The Worst of Kalaki

and

The Best of Yuss

Script by Roy Clarke

Animation by Trevor Ford

Published by Bookworld Publishers
PO Box 32581, Lusaka, Zambia
2004

Copyright text © *The Post* 2004
Copyright Illustrations © Trevor Ford 2004

All rights reserved. No part of this publication may be reproduced, stored in a retrieval system, or transmitted, in any form or by any means electronic, mechanical, photocopying, recording or otherwise, without the prior permission of the publisher.

ISBN 9982-24-031-5

Typesetting by Fergan Limited, Lusaka, Zambia
Printing by Intrepid Printers (Pty) Ltd
8147

Dedicated to the memory of

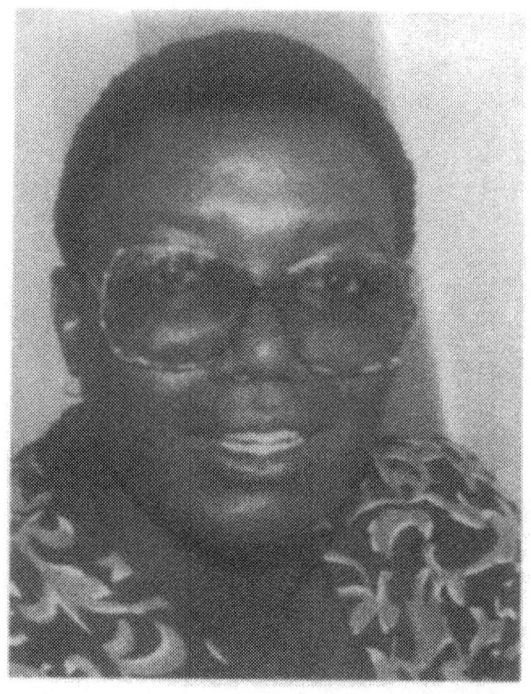

Lucy Sichone

Champion of Press Freedom

Contents

Chapter	Article	Page
Preface		ix
1. Mfuwe and Back		**1**
	1.1 Mfuwe	2
	1.2 Baboon	5
	1.3 The Last Laugh	7
	1.4 Upside Down	10
	1.5 Shikashiwa	12
	1.6 Back to Mfuwe	14
	1.7 The Lawnmower	16
2. Kings and Things		**19**
	2.1 Kanono's Diary	20
	2.2 Haunted House	23
	2.3 Unity	26
	2.4 The Palace	28
	2.5 The Red Carpet	30
	2.6 Indaba Maningi	32
3. Thoko's Teddy		**34**
	3.1 King Kanono	35
	3.2 Swallowed	38
	3.3 Thoko's Teddy	40
	3.4 Zoo Story	42
	3.5 Up and Down	44
	3.6 The Plunderer	46
4. Mumbo Jumbo		**49**
	4.1 Never!	50
	4.2 Mumbo Jumbo	52
	4.3 God's Plan	55
	4.4 Voice of Vice	57
	4.5 Saved!	59
5. Wabufi Kafupi		**62**
	5.1 Forgive me, Father...	63

5.2 Letter from the Bahamas	65
5.3 Paramount Thief	68
5.4 The Settlement	70
5.5 The Chosen One	72
5.6 Sheriff's Sale	74
5.7 Vera's Story	76
5.8 Death Trap	78
6. Vera's Diary	**80**
6.1 The Auction	81
6.2 All is not Lost!	84
6.3 Flee at Last!	86
6.4 The Gleen Libbon	88
6.5 The Exorcist	90
7. Third Term Madness	**92**
7.1 The Official Candidate	93
7.2 False Pretences	95
7.3 Hippomania	98
7.4 Gospel Truth	100
7.5 Ratification	102
7.6 Rising to the Occasion	104
7.7 Follow the Rules	106
7.8 The Presidential Candidate	108
8. Elections and Erections	**110**
8.1 Road to Manda Hill	111
8.2 The Silly Ass	113
8.3 Super Salesman	116
8.4 Dr Freddistein's Monster	118
8.5 The Bus	120
8.6 Nomination Day	122
8.7 Election Race	124
8.8 A New Leaf	127
8.9 Employment Opportunity	129
9. Religiously Irreligious	**131**
9.1 St Ignominious	132
9.2 An Extraordinary Death	134
9.3 Prayer for the Departed	137
9.4 Resurrection	139

	9.5 Free Willy	141
10. Strange Encounters		**143**
	10.1 Mr Forgettable	144
	10.2 Sir Frantic	146
	10.3 Popular Choice	148
	10.4 Strange Encounter	150
	10.5 Cherise	152
	10.6 Bloodsuckers	154
	10.7 Professor Supple	156
11. Contempt of Court		**159**
	11.1 The Merry Judge	160
	11.2 Where is it?	163
	11.3 The Trough	165
	11.4 The Cookie Monster	167

Note:
The date of publication of each article in *The Post* may be found at the foot of each article.

Preface

Early this year a dark cloud of deportation hung over the head of *Post* columnist, Roy Clarke. Shortly after the publication of his piece entitled *Mfuwe*, the government declared that Roy was a 'threat to peace and good order', and ordered his deportation from Zambia, a country where he has lived for the past forty-two years.

While his lawyer was bringing the matter to court, and while the security services were searching for him, Roy went into hiding. By the time he emerged, he had revealed himself as an uncompromising champion of the freedom of the press, and of freedom of expression in general. He had refused to make any apology, and instead continued issuing his trenchant weekly column from his 'spider hole'. He was prepared to be deported rather than enter into compromises that might encroach upon the freedom of the press, and make the work of his fellow Zambian journalists even more difficult.

As a writer, Roy has developed his own style of satire as a means for social and political criticism. In this, he has continued and developed the satirical tradition of Kapelwa Musonda, who wrote for many years in the *Times*. His work can also be seen as an outgrowth from the more direct style of political criticism practised by the late lamented Lucy Sichone and Jowie Mwinga. Roy has utilised the space carved out by these previous exponents, and may even be credited with using his own sharp pen to enlarge that space a bit further.

In his *Spectator* column, Roy holds up a mirror wherein beholders do generally discover everybody's face but their own. And so we can understand why some people feel so offended by Roy's literary works. They find it easy to recognise others, and laugh at them. But they cannot laugh at themselves! The ability to laugh at yourself is a rare talent, but it is essential for any person with ambitions to enter public life.

It is not easy to write the way Roy does. Roy is a master of the English language, using irony, sarcasm and caustic wit to expose human folly, vice, and hypocrisy. This, by definition, is the project of satire. He aims to expose the ridiculous in individuals, organisations or institutions. Recent public reaction to his writing is testimony to the extent that he has succeeded in attracting attention. It simply can't be ignored. And this is the way it should be, provocative, to demand attention, to provoke thought and the demand for change. Of what value would it be if it were simply ignored?

Our country should take pride in its critics, and especially in creative critics like Roy. Until we can allow our people the fullest and unencumbered expression in art, writing and politics, we are in danger of presenting a very simplified and one-dimensional view of this complex universe.

A society without critics is a human hell where leaders may indulge their dictatorial instincts without moral compunction. Some people claim that criticism of our leaders is alien to our custom and tradition. They forget that in our traditional past even chiefs or kings were the subject of satirical orations, through poetry and ribaldry, often presented to their face. By such means, even the ruthless Shaka Zulu could be openly criticised.

But nowadays, just try to criticise or ridicule the president of this country and see what happens to you! Some people are very fond of justifying our political practices in terms of our ancestral traditions, even when they are actually very ignorant of these traditions.

Nowadays we find ourselves stuck in a culture of zealous worship of leaders, a culture that would look primitive in the eyes of our ancestors. Our modern African societies have established a reputation for intolerance that is difficult to match. In this suffocating political environment, people lose the habit of thinking, let alone exchanging creative views and thoughts. This is not the African culture of our ancestors, but a twisted version that is corrupt, crude and cruel.

I see Roy's work as attempting to confront this situation, to help us return to our more tolerant Zambian culture; a culture of liberating, life-giving and enjoyable laughter!

Fred M'membe.
Editor of *The Post*.   2nd June 2004

Chapter 1
Mfuwe and Back

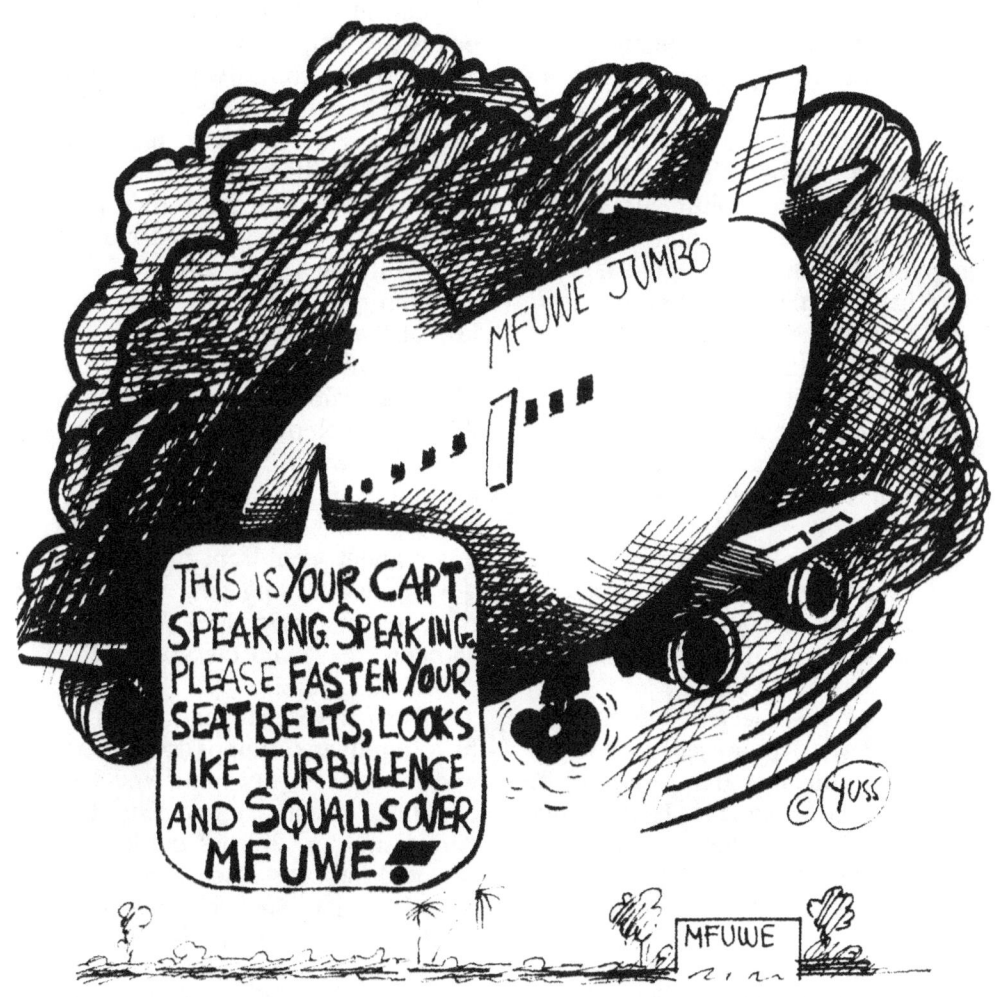

1.1 Mfuwe

HE lumbered out of the state lodge, staggered towards the massive wooden chair that had been made ready for him, and fell backwards into it. His dishevelled safari suit was unbuttoned, and his huge belly hung over his trousers. In front of him sat all the assembled animals of Mfuwe, waiting for the Great Elephant Muwelewele to begin his Christmas Message.

'Distinguished elephants, honourable hippos, mischievous monkeys, parasitic politicians, bureaucratic buffaloes, and other anonymous animals,' he began, 'I have just returned from one of my very brief visits to Lusaka, in order to be with you at this time of celebration. My message to you is that the last year has been a resounding economic success, and Mfuwe has never been more prosperous!'

'Ee ee eeyee,' squealed the monkeys, dancing around in circles, and waggling their bottoms, each painted with a picture of the Great Elephant.

'When I was elected,' continued Muwelewele, 'I promised that only those constituencies that voted for me would see development. That is why Mfuwe is the only constituency that has seen development.'

'Iwe wakhonza!' shouted the crowd.

'All the humans in the rest of this country refused to vote for me, so they have had no share in our marvellous development!'

'Chabwino!' shouted the crowd.

'It was only you, my friends from the game park, who went out there and brought in twenty-nine percent of the vote. The snakes of the Shushushu slithered into the ballot boxes and stuffed them with votes. The horrible hyenas were our trusted party cadres who chased away the opposition voters. Our reliable rhinos moved the polling stations to unknown places in the forest. And our merry monkeys played hide and seek with the voters cards!'

'Hurray!' laughed the crowd. 'The law of the jungle!'

'So now the MMD is the Movement for Mfuwe Development. All my development programmes are located in Mfuwe, and all my appointments have been from amongst you. The previous government would not put you in government, saying you were just monkeys and crocodiles, who shouldn't be given the vote.'

'Chamanyazi!'

'But I have changed all that. I have nominated hippos to parliament, and made them my ministers! I have appointed jackals as my district administrators, and put the long-fingered baboons in charge of the treasury. I have put the knock-kneed giraffe in charge of agriculture, the hungry crocodile in charge of child welfare, and the red-lipped snake in

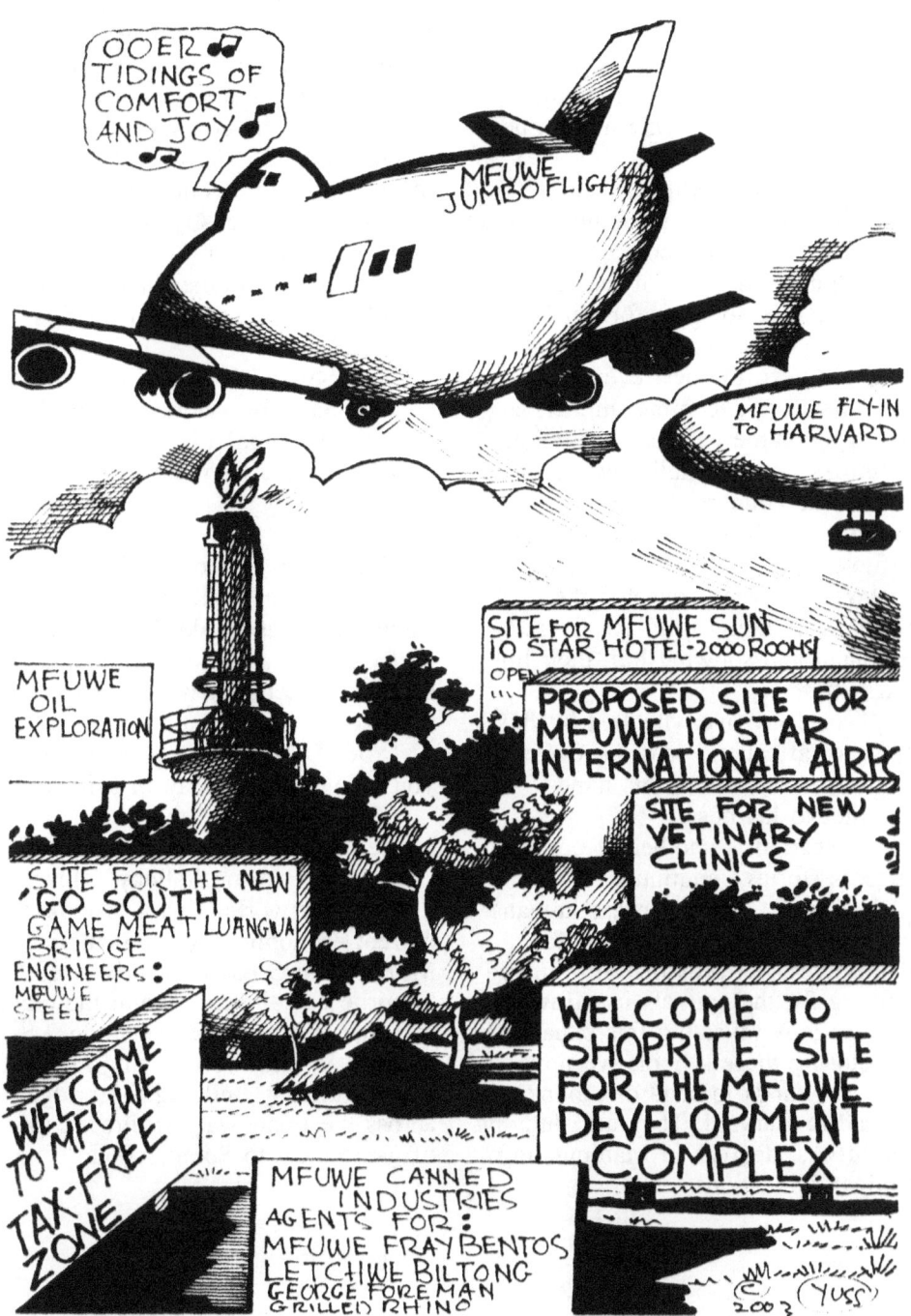

charge of legal reform. And best of all, the pythons are now fully employed, squeezing the taxpayers!'

'One family one government!' cheered the crowd. 'One hippo one minister!'

'Our beloved Mfuwe,' said Muwelewele solemnly, 'is now a state within the state. We control everything in the rest of the country. Everything is now run for our benefit. I am pleased to report that the past year has been the best ever. Just as the others are becoming thinner, so we in the game park are becoming fatter. As hospitals fall down in the rest of the country, so we are building veterinary clinics all over Mfuwe.'

'Wehwehweh!' squeeled the baboons, running up to the Great Elephant and showing him their big red bottoms.

'I am truly overwhelmed by this show of affection,' said the Great Muwelewele, holding his hand-kerchief to his nose.

'Education is another of our great success stories,' continued Muwelewele. 'The heartless humans built schools and universities for themselves, but provided absolutely nothing for the animals in Mfuwe. We are now reversing this situation. By closing these schools we now have the funds to send our monkeys abroad to Harvard. They are studying for MBAs, degrees in Manipulating Budget Allocations.

'Just as employment is falling rapidly amongst the humans, so it is increasing rapidly here in Mfuwe. Just as factories are closing in the remainder of the country, so they are increasing here. I have declared Mfuwe a tax-free zone, and our new manufacturing industry will soon be exporting directly to South Africa. A new bridge across the Luangwa is already under construction for this purpose.'

'Our Saviour,' shouted the crowd. 'A new Saviour is born! A New Deal! A New Direction! Let's roast a few street kids, and have a real feast!'

The jumbo glided to a halt at Lusaka International Airport. Out came the Great Leader Muwelewele, lumbering down the steps like an elephant. A reporter managed to thrust a microphone in front of him.

'Your Divine Majesty, how did you enjoy your holiday in Mfuwe?'

'What!' exploded the Great Leader, his face turning purple with rage. 'I was not on holiday! This was a very busy working trip, to look at current economic developments in Mfuwe, which has been privatised. Shoprite has already bought the place, and they are busy putting in an abattoir and meat processing factory. We are already building the bridge across the Luangwa, for direct export of game meat to South Africa!'

1st January 2004

1.2   Baboon

THE King was in his palace, sitting on his throne, reading the morning papers. In the corner sat a whiskery baboon of a fellow, scribbling on his notepad. The silence was interrupted by a timid knock on the door. 'Come in!' boomed the King, as a giant of a man lumbered in, more like a dinosaur, of the sort generally thought to be extinct. It was the dreaded Shaky Shikashiwa, Minister of Law and Disorder.

'You asked to see me, Your Majesty?' said the Minister, bowing very low.

'Yes!' roared the King, 'What are these dreadful things I've been hearing about you? I've called you here to explain yourself!'

'I can't think what you might mean, Your Most Divine Majesty,' replied Shikashiwa, attempting to humble himself with a wobbly grovel.

'Well you'd better start thinking fast,' snapped the King, 'if its not too late in your career. Do you see who that is, sitting in the corner?'

'Looks more like a baboon to me. Did you bring him from Mfuwe?'

'There's no need to make animalistic remarks,' said the baboon. 'I happen to be descended from a long line of hairy ancestors. I am Spectacle Kalaliki, the one who digs deeper for *The Boast*.'

'Ha ha!' shouted the Mighty Shikashiwa, lurching forward, 'My policee have been searching for him all week!'

'Not so fast!' commanded the King, 'Stay where you are and don't touch him! He is staying here under my protection. He has been telling me that you have called him a baboon, accused him of defaming the government, and you are trying to deport him to Mfuwe..'

'My dear brother, let me explain...'

'Don't you call me your brother!' screamed the King. 'People will think that's your only qualification for the job!'

'My deepest apologies Your Majesty. You see the problem arose when your nephew...'

'My nephew!' screamed the King. 'What sort of talk is this? Doesn't he have a name?'

'Sorry Your Majesty. I mean Mr Putrid Bumble, my Executive Secretary. He got terribly upset when Kalaliki wrote a story about hippos. Apparently the story included one particularly fat hippo which he immediately recognised as himself.'

'He should get his weight down,' snapped the King, 'if he wants to avoid such confusion of identity. But you, Shikashiwa, how did you get into all this?'

'I was coming to that, Your Majesty. The first I knew about it was when there was a rumpus outside my office. Apparently Putrid Bumble had gone into Wachama and rented a gang of kaponya to demand the blood of Kalaliki, and I had to go out there and face this bloodthirsty mob. They were already carrying Kalaliki's coffin, in readiness for the dreadful deed.'

'That's right,' interrupted Kalaliki, looking up from his notepad. 'That's when I came running to the palace for protection.'

The King turned towards the hapless Shikashiwa. 'But aren't you the very one who should have given him protection?'

'Oh I did, Your Majesty. To protect him from the murderous mob, I promised to deport him to Mfuwe. After all, he's obviously a baboon, so that's where he must have originated.'

'Try to get baboons out from your mind,' growled the King. 'What you were supposed to have done was to tell the mob that murder carries the death penalty. And also that you had to follow the rule of law. If Bumble had been defamed, then his proper remedy is to go before a judge to complain, and explain how he had managed to identify himself as the hippo in the story written by Kalaliki. Shikashiwa, don't you understand the smallest thing about government policy?'

'Oh yes, Your Majesty. That's why I have all the policee out looking for Kalaliki.'

'Not police!' screamed the King. 'I'm talking about policy. My government is supposed to stand for the rule of law and freedom of the press. Look at all these newspapers,' he said, sweeping his hand towards the pile on the table. 'I have the international press and human rights organisations from all over the world on my neck! This little Kalaliki is becoming famous, while your Great King is becoming infamous!'

'Terribly sorry, Your Majesty. You must tell me how this new policee is different from our old policee. Do they wear different uniforms?'

'I am going to give you time to find out. I am sending both you and Bumble on forced leave for six months!'

'Where should we go, Your Most Divine Majesty?'

'To Mfuwe,' declared the King.

As the door closed behind the Minister, the King turned to Kalaliki. 'I hope you won't report all this in tomorrow's paper.'

'Its out of my hands,' said Kalaliki. 'That's entirely for the Editor to decide.'

7th January 2004

1.3 The Last Laugh

'GRANDPA,' said Thoko, 'Me and Kondwa want a story before we go to bed.'

'Once upon a time,' I began, 'a very long time ago in the faraway land of Nseko, there lived the great King Muwelewele.'

'Muwelewele?' said Kondwa, 'what does that mean?'

'It means a very clever and wise person,' I explained.

'And the people of Nseko,' suggested Thoko, 'were very fond of laughing at everything.'

'That's right,' I laughed. 'Nseko was the most marvellous place, for laughter is the voice of the Gods, come down here on Earth to visit us. For its only laughter that makes us human.'

'Huh,' said Kondwa, 'animals also laugh!'

'No they don't,' laughed Thoko. 'An elephant trumpets, a lion roars, a bird tweets, a mouse squeaks and a monkey chatters...'

'Monkeys laugh,' said Kondwa.

'Monkeys don't laugh,' I said sternly. 'They can only chortle, usually over trivial matters such as stealing somebody else's nuts. This is merely evil glee, nothing like our sense of humour.'

'Look Grandpa,' said Thoko, 'never mind Kondwa, can you just get on with the story? If it's a story, something is supposed to happen!'

'Yes,' I gulped. 'I was coming to that. An awful thing happened. The Great King Muwelewele was out riding one day when he had a terrible accident, and fell off his horse.'

'Why did he fall off his horse?' demanded Kondwa.

'The horse saw the dreaded red-lipped snake, and reared up into the air in fright, and the king was thrown to the ground, landing on his head.'

'He lost his brains,' said Kondwa.

'No, it was worse than that,' I said, 'he lost his sense of humour. He was supposed to be king of all Nseko, but after the accident he couldn't laugh and he couldn't stand other people laughing. He thought they were all laughing at him. He made a Deportation Order that all laughter was to be deported from the land.'

'Oh dear,' said Thoko. 'Wasn't that against the Constootion.'

'Exactly,' I said. 'In those days constootions were always very small. Nseko had just one small piece of paper with the words *Every citizen is free to laugh.*'

'So he was being unconstititootional,' insisted Thoko.

'He altered the constootion,' I explained. 'Now it read *Every citizen is free to laugh, after he has been deported.*'

'But he couldn't deport everybody,' said Thoko.

'Exactly,' I said. 'So he employed the Director of Unicef, Dr Serious Going, to vaccinate everybody against laughing.'

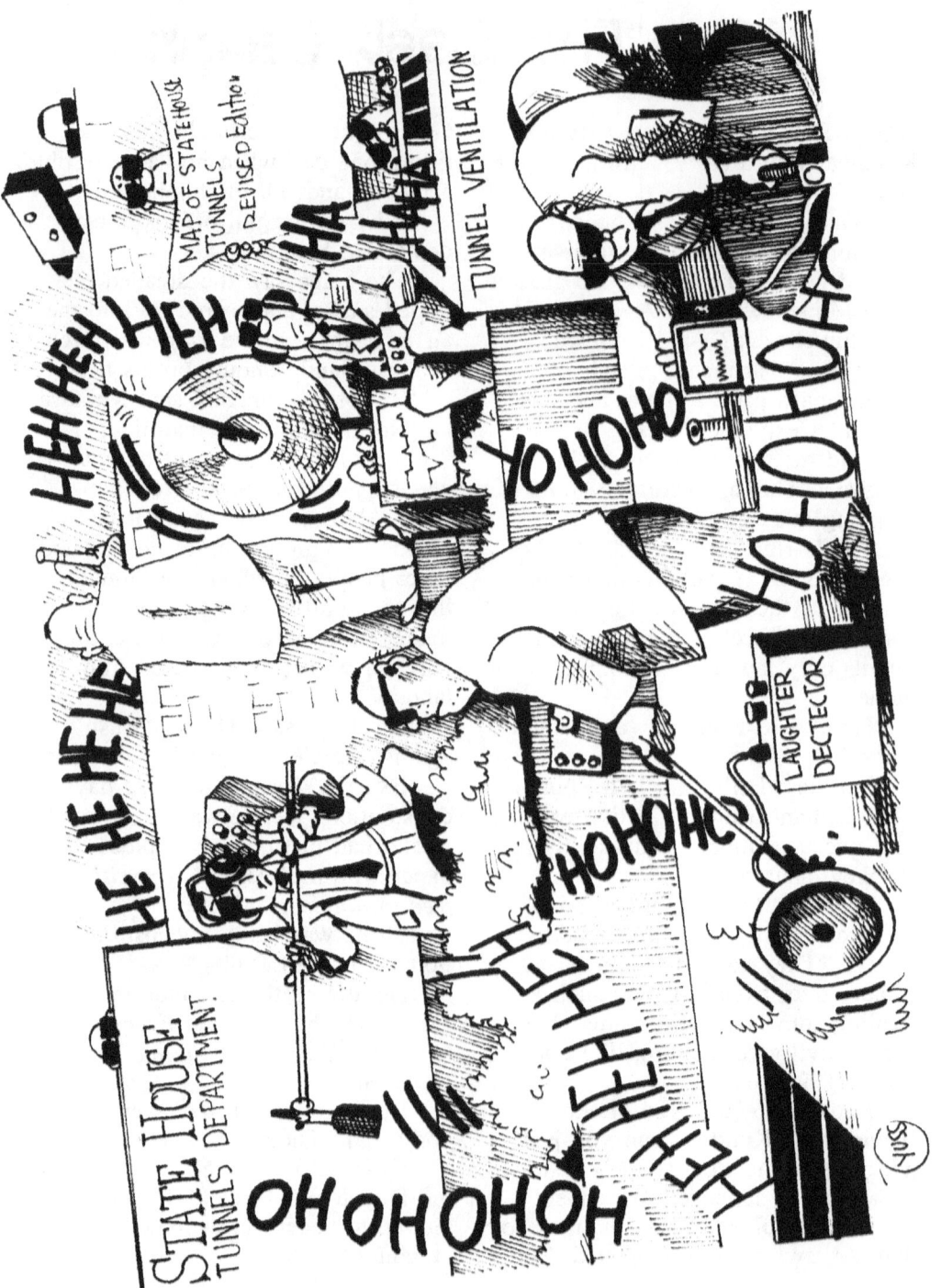

'Laughing is not a disease,' said Kondwa.

'Oh yes it is,' snapped Thoko. 'Its extremely infectious.'

'And did Serious Going manage to vaccinate everybody?' asked Kondwa.

'It was very Serious Going indeed,' I said. 'She managed to catch everybody except the notorious Cackling Kalaki, who went into hiding.'

'Where did he hide?' asked Thoko.

'He hid in the drains, and in the sewers, and in the cellars. And all the King's horses and all the King's men couldn't find him. But all the time they could hear him laughing, and they thought he was laughing at them. The King flew into a terrible rage when he heard the cacophonous cackle of Cackling Kalaki coming up from the tunnels under his palace. He could hear him but he couldn't find him.'

'He wouldn't give himself up?'

'He couldn't. For the Gods had given him the sacred task of protecting the Last Laugh. If he lost it, everything would be lost. But while he was down there, he had an idea. And so he invented something quite new.'

'Huh,' said Kondwa. 'What was that?'

'He spent all his time flattening and polishing a metal plate, and by so doing he made the first ever mirror. But he had also invented a new form of laughter. He had realised that if people could see themselves as they really are, they would have to laugh. And this would be a new type of laughter, more noble and more hilarious. And it would be a new strain of laughter that could not be killed by Unicef vaccination.

'So one day he rose up out of a manhole in the middle of the market, looked at himself in the mirror, and started laughing like a maniac. Other people immediately grabbed the mirror to look in it, to see what was funny. And they also started laughing, with a very infectious laugh. Before long the whole nation was laughing, and Nseko was reborn! For when people are able to laugh at themselves, that is the highest level of civilisation!'

'But what about the King?' asked Kondwa. 'He couldn't laugh.'

'Even the King,' I said, 'as soon as he looked in the mirror he found his long-lost sense of humour. It had been hiding in the mirror! *Ha ha,* laughed the King, *I look just like an elephant!*'

'But you said elephants can't laugh!' said Kondwa.

'They can't,' said Thoko. 'So that just shows that he wasn't really an elephant!'

15th January 2004

1.4 Upside Down

'WHERE are you off to this morning?' I asked Kupela, as she swept past me, hair flying and bangles jangling.

'Professor Muchenjelo's lecture on satire,' said Koops. 'You should come along, you might learn something.'

'I'm too old to be a student.'

'They still have the tradition that anybody can drop in, a hangover from when it was the People's University.'

An hour later we were sitting at the back of the crammed lecture hall, as the famous Professor Muchenjelo swept in, wearing a purple frock. On his head was a lovely shiny green fez, with a gold tassle hanging down over his face.

'This morning's lecture,' he said, as he took a bright red book out of his pink handbag, 'is about satire. All you need to know about satire is contained in the piece I am about to read.'

He opened the book slowly, found the page, and began to read. 'The wise King Muwelewele ruled over a pleasant and friendly land. The King himself was much loved, for he was very generous to all his friends and relatives, appointing them as his ministers.

'But one day a terrible thing happened. The King put on his spectacles upside down. With the result that he saw the whole world upside down. *Ah ha!* exclaimed the King, *I have been looking for a New Vision for my country. Now the Lord has enabled me to see things differently, so I can go down in history as a Wise King.*

'So the King immediately summoned parliament to make a speech about his New Vision. But just as he was about to begin his speech, he turned to one of the twenty-six security officers standing behind him, hissing at him, *There's nobody on the floor of the House, they're all on the ceiling. Do they think they're higher than me, their King, who was appointed by God! This is treason!*

'*Do not worry, Your Most Marvellous Majesty,* replied the security officer, *This just means that their ideas are all in the air, and that you are the only one with your feet on the ground.*

'*Quite right,* said the King, as he began his speech. *Most Honourable Paid Puppets of Parliament, I have come here today to give you my New Vision. I have this morning discovered that until now our whole world has been upside down. But now I have a vision for putting it the right way up.*

'*Hurray!* they all cheered, so loudly that they nearly fell off the ceiling.

'*Firstly, our transport system has been upside down. In future, to avoid potholes, all motorcars will fly, and only aeroplanes will use the roads.*

'*I am also changing the system of*

law, so that all people will be deemed guilty until proven innocent. Only innocent people will go to jail, and the guilty shall be set free. The judges who sent them to jail must make confessions, and bow down low before convicted murderers.

'And so the Rule of Law will be replaced by the Rule of Roar, where the innocent will be punished according to the loudness of the Roar from a drunken mob of hired thugs.

'Hurray! cheered the House of Parliamentary Puppets, *'This is what we mean by democracy!'*

Now the Great Professor looked up from his text and addressed the students directly. 'This story,' he said, 'is a paradigm example of satire. What, I ask you, is the true meaning of this story?'

'It means,' suggested one student, 'that the King should consult others before trying to change things.'

'Hum,' replied Professor Muchenjelo, 'but surely a King is guided by God, and does not need to consult mere mortals!'

'It is a warning,' said another student, 'against taking decisions too hastily, on the basis of insufficient evidence and reasoning. The King should have realised that it was his spectacles that were upside down, and not the whole country!'

'But have you considered,' replied the Great Professor, 'these might have been magic spectacles which gave the King an entirely new theoretical perspective on the problems facing the country!'

'So tell us, Great Professor, what does it really mean?'

'What it really means,' shouted Muchenjelo, 'is that this writer insulted the King, and for this crime he was executed. What it also means to you students is that you must not question higher authorities. You should just write down what I say and memorise it for the exam. Anybody found writing anything satirical about me will be expelled!'

'That's you,' Kupela whispered in my ear. 'You've been expelled already!'

'He's got a very peculiar voice,' I said, 'it sounds as if he is squeezing it out from between his cheeks.'

'Have you only just realised,' laughed Kupela, 'that he's been talking through his rear end.'

'You mean he's upside down?'

'Exactly,' said Kupela.

22nd January 2004

1.5 Shikashiwa

'AH ha, Spectator Kalaki!' he said, rising from his desk to greet me, 'how nice to meet you.'

'It is my privilege,' I said, as we shook hands, 'to meet the famous Shaky Shikashiwa, Minister for Absurdity and Hilarity. What can I do for you?'

'Well,' he said, 'I've been following your satire, and I thought perhaps you could advise me in my national duty of making the whole nation laugh.'

'Is this the New Direction we've all been waiting for?'

'Its the only one we've got!' he laughed. 'What with the AIDS crisis and grinding poverty, we need everybody to keep laughing, or they might get cross with the government.'

'But are you properly qualified to make people laugh? Some people say you were only appointed because you're the King's uncle!'

A slight frown crossed his face. 'That's not true,' he said, as he stood up from his chair, drawing himself up to his full height of two metres. 'Look at me, am I not truly monstrous and ridiculous in my own right?'

'You are indeed,' I agreed. 'When did you first learn to make people laugh?'

'At school,' he replied, 'where the only skill I acquired was the ability to fall flat on my face. It always provoked gales of laughter. And that's how,' he laughed, 'I developed this huge misshapen nose.'

It certainly was a Guinness Record nose, looking more like a purple cabbage. 'That's a considerable asset,' I admitted, 'if you want to make people laugh. But have you made your career entirely by falling flat on your face?'

'Recently I have been trying to develop more subtle alternatives. After reading your work, I have been trying to move the government in the New Direction of satire. You know, making people laugh at the serious things in life, such as democracy and the constitution.'

'That's more like it,' I said, 'and less damaging to the nose! What's your current satirical project?'

'Come and see,' he said, taking me by the hand, and walking me to the window. There below us in the street was a mob of drunken thugs carrying a black coffin with the word *Democracy* written on the side.

'What's funny about that?' I asked.

'Don't you see?' he laughed. 'Our government stands for democracy, but we are being asked by this mindless mob to murder it, and bury it! Hilarious!'

'It will certainly make people think!'

'Exactly. This is not merely hilarious. This is the theatre of the absurd, which has a deeper purpose. It is designed to provoke ordinary citizens to see the dangers of mob rule.'

'But where did these drunken thugs come from?'

'They're really actors, employed by the government.'

'Even so, aren't the police supposed to move in to protect democracy?'

'Those are also not really the police. They're just party cadres dressed up in police uniforms. The whole point of this street theatre is to see if ordinary people will have the courage to move in and protect democracy, even when the government seems to be doing nothing about it. Therefore this scene, which is apparently just hilarious on its surface, has a deeper implication for civic education and popular action to prevent dictatorship.'

'Splendid,' I said. 'What other marvellous satirical theatre have you devised?'

'We had great fun at the High Court the other day, when I employed a court jester, dressed up as a lawyer, to demand an undertaking from the Judge that I have absolute powers in all my buffoonery. I sought a ruling that my absurdities cannot be constrained by the court. My jester even ripped out the section on the *Independence of the Judiciary* from the Constitution, tore it into pieces, and threw it in the face of the Judge!'

'So what was the result?'

'Everybody laughed so much that the case was laughed out of court. As a result, the *Independence of the Judiciary* and *Separation of Powers* have now been strengthened. In his ruling the Judge made it clear that the jester's arguments were absurd and hilarious. This just shows how satire can contribute to good governance.'

Just then the phone rang, and Shikashiwa picked it up. 'Yes, Your Majesty,' he said. 'Very sorry, Your Majesty ... I do understand, Your Majesty.'

As he put the phone down, the laughable Shikashiwa had suddenly stopped laughing. The bags of flab on his huge comical face now sagged down into an enormous sadness, and a tear ran down his face.

'My dear fellow,' I said, 'what on earth has happened?'

'That was the Great King Muwelewele. He was not amused by the mob of thugs outside his palace, demanding his deportation. I've been fired!'

'Some people,' I said, 'just haven't got a sense of humour.'

'Its all your fault, Kalaki,' sobbed Shikashiwa. 'If it hadn't been for your satire, I'd never have gotten into this mess.'

29th January 2004

1.6 Back to Mfuwe

ALL the animals were seated in a great half circle as Bloated Nsofu Makangi stood up to address the Mfuwe National Assembly...

'Mister Unspeakable, Sir,' began Makangi, 'as his Elephant for Squandering, the Great Elephant Muwelewele has sent me here to present his Budget for 2004.

'First I should explain to this august House that all our squandering in the previous year of 2003 was extremely successful, with squandering exceeding extortion by over 300 per cent!'

'Hurray!' trumpeted the elephants. 'Praise the Great Squanderer!'

'Moreover,' continued Makangi, 'for much of this squandering we must be grateful to Our Great Leader Muwelewele. During the past year he managed to travel to 43 different countries in his search of his *New Vision* for our beautiful country. Our Great Leader has also promised to bring us the *Rule of Law*, so it is crucially important that he travels to many different countries to try to find out what these wonderful words might mean.'

This praise of the Great Leader provoked a trumpeting chant from all the assembled elephants,

All animals are equal,
But elephants are power.
Born to wander,
Born to squander,
Elephants are power!

'Exactly,' said Nsofu Makangi. 'We must understand that we are not elephants because we have power, but we have power because we are elephants!'

'Nonsense! Point of Order!' squealed the monkeys. 'You are elephants because you eat too much. If we had power, we would also be elephants!'

'This is a wrong perception of democracy which has caused so much trouble in the past,' declared Makangi. 'You monkeys have been misled by socialism, foolishly imagining that if you get educated, then you could get power and become elephants.'

Again the elephants began to trumpet,

All elephants are educated,
But not all educated are elephants.
Education means power,
Power for the elephants.

'Exactly,' said Makangi. 'Monkeys and even crocodiles have been educating themselves, thinking they could become elephants. This is a complete misconception. In this Budget I propose to save funds by closing down all government schools and universities.'

'What!' squealed the monkeys. 'What about education for all?'

'According to government policy, education has now been privatised. It is now the private responsibility of parents to send their offspring to private schools. In this way, monkeys will be brought up as monkeys, and not imagine that they can grow into elephants.'

'What happened to the government of the people?' squealed the monkeys.

'This is now a new era,' said Makangi solemnly. 'Government of the elephant, by the elephant, for the elephant. Therefore the Education Budget now becomes an Education Allowance for Elephants. Obviously we can't waste the government budget on people who have no hope of getting into government.'

'So what is the government going to be doing for us?'

'Ask not what your government can do for you, but ask what you can do for your government! For example, the government has been spending huge sums on hospitals and clinics, but you monkeys are spreading cholera out of carelessness and negligence, and spreading HIV on purpose. How can the government help you if you are refusing to help yourselves?'

'So is the Health Budget also cancelled?'

'Not at all. In the past, we elephants had to spend huge amounts of money trekking to South Africa for medical attention. This was because we did not dare to visit government hospitals that were full of unhygienic patients, and infested with rats, cockroaches, mosquitoes and fleas. The patients were so diseased that the nurses refused to touch them, and all the doctors fled abroad. In future government facilities will be reserved for government, and private facilities reserved for private citizens. That is what we mean by privatisation.'

'Then why should we pay taxes, if all the money goes to you?'

'It is a basic principle of equality that all animals must give according to their ability, and receive according to their need. It is in the nature of things that monkeys and baboons are very active at collecting food, but do not need much. We elephants, on the other hand, can only move very slowly, in order to maintain our great dignity, but we need enormous quantities of food. This is why I am calling this an Activity Budget. We must tax the active to feed the inactive.'

'No!' screamed the monkeys. 'We shall never pass this Budget.'

'Because of the increased cost of Our Great Leader's foreign travel,' persisted Makangi, 'I am proposing that Income Tax be raised to 50%, and Vicious Addition Tax to 30%.'

'Never!' screamed the monkeys. 'Over our dead bodies!'

'And with the additional revenue,' Makangi continued calmly, 'I intend to increase sitting allowance to a million gluders a day, and car loans to a billion gluders!'

'That's more like it!' squealed the monkeys. 'Budget approved! Long live the Great Elephant Muwelewele!'

4th January 2004

1.7 The Lawnmower

I cycled in through the iron gates of Chikwa Magistrates Court at exactly eight o'clock, the time stipulated on the police bond. I had expected the police to be waiting for me, to take me back into their custody, but the place was deserted.

I parked my bike in the garage, and walked towards the front door. I sat down on an ancient rusty lawnmower parked next to an overgrown bush. On it, moulded into the cast iron, were the words *Birmingham 1942*. Strange coincidence, I thought. I was also made in Birmingham in 1942. Now we were here together again, both disintegrating.

'Good morning,' said a voice behind me, making me jump. I turned round to find a grey old man. 'I'm Oloso Zulu,' he said, 'The caretaker.'

'I'm Kalaki,' I replied, standing up to greet him. 'Oloso? The name rings a bell. Didn't you used to be somebody?'

'Even you oloso,' he laughed, 'you used to be somebody.'

'Is this old motor mower still working?' I asked.

'Of course not,' he laughed. 'It's obsolete colonial technology. As soon as we got into power we set up the National Council for Scientific Research, which invented the slasher.'

The old boy went whistling happily away amongst the ruins of his courtroom, as I stood there, leaning against the high metal handle of the lawnmower, wondering whether I would be able to make a success of life in prison. But my ambitious plans for the future were interrupted by another voice. 'Muli bwanji, Ba Kalaki!'

Again I looked round, but couldn't see anybody.

'I am down here, Ba Kalaki!'

I looked down, and there was my little friend Kafupi. 'Wabufi!' I cried, shaking his hand, and sitting on the lawnmower to get down to his level. 'I haven't seen you for ages! Have you come to observe my court case?'

A slight frown crossed his brow. 'I thought you'd come to see mine! What are you charged with?'

'Two counts of trying to encourage a policeman to do his duty.'

'That's very serious,' he laughed. 'If a policeman rushes off to do his duty he could easily get hurt, or get his uniform dirty.'

'And interfere with people's basic freedoms,' I suggested.

'Exactly,' said Kafupi. 'Like that rampage of MMD thugs outside the Supreme Court the other day. They were exercising their freedom of movement and freedom of expression. In the interest of democracy the police refused to interfere!'

Just then a busload of people drove into the yard. 'Ah Ha!' exclaimed Kafupi, 'my supporters are here at last!'

Fifty people unloaded from the bus and began shouting 'Kalaki! Kalaki!',

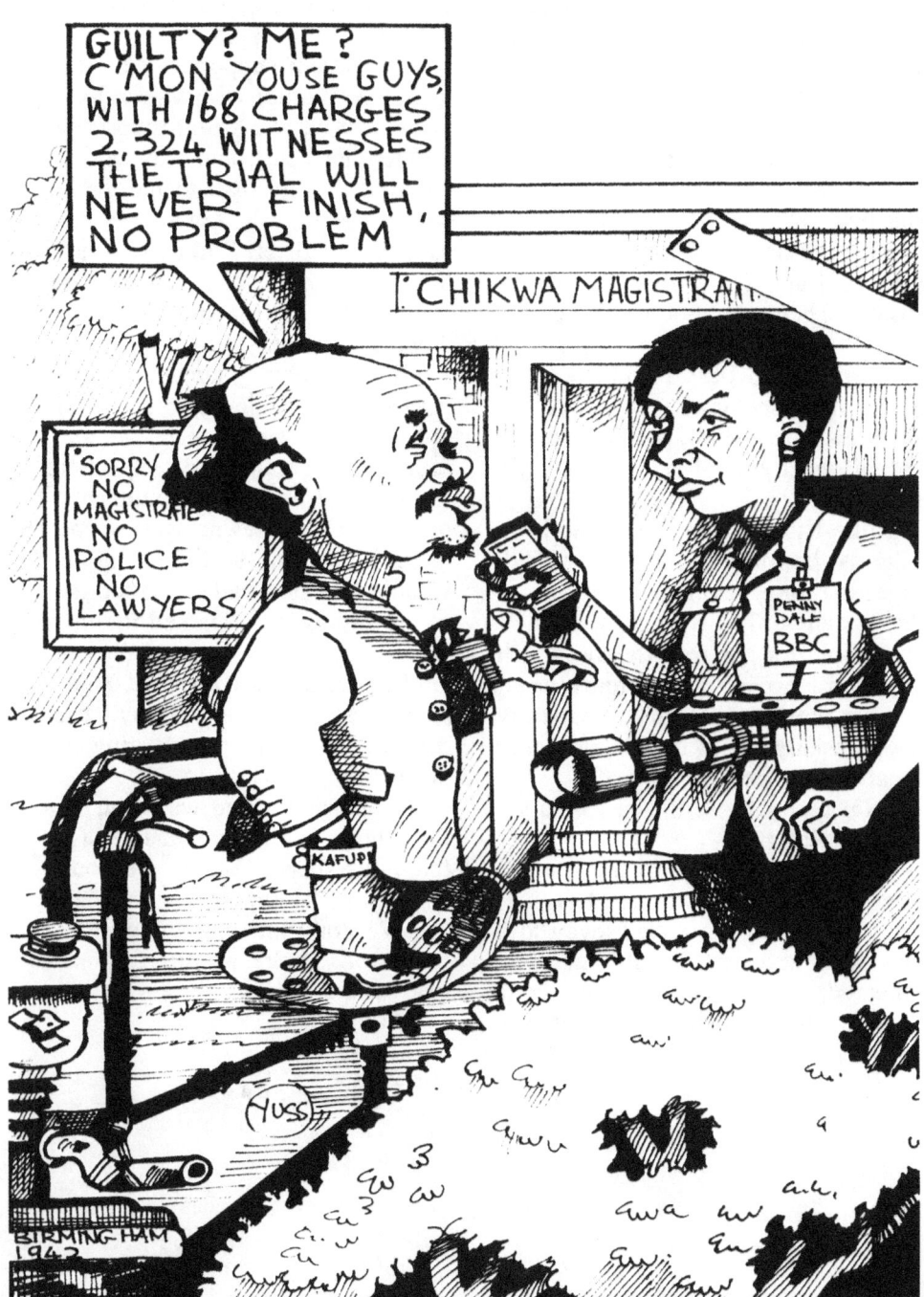

and then came over to shake hands with both of us. Then up came Penny Dale from the BBC, microphone outstretched. 'What sort of sentence are you expecting, Kalaki?'

'I've got two charges,' I explained, 'so I expect two deportation orders. The first order will deport me from Lusaka to London. Then the second order will deport me from London to Lusaka. Then everybody will be happy!'

Then I lifted little Kafupi onto the lawnmower, so that Penny could interview him. 'Well, Mr Wabufi Kafupi, what sort of sentence are you expecting?'

Little Kafupi grew bigger and taller as the microphone was pushed under his nose. 'Well, with 168 charges and 2,324 witnesses, it is impossible for the trial to ever finish. So I don't expect any sentence at all.'

'Not you,' said Penny impatiently. 'I was asking about the Kalaki case. What verdict do you expect?'

'Not guilty by virtue of insanity,' laughed Kafupi.

Just then the Clerk of the Court came out and spoke to us. 'The magistrate has been called away to a funeral, none of the lawyers have appeared, and the police cannot come because of lack of transport. The court hearing is therefore adjourned until 26 March 2005.'

The Kalaki supporters got back in their bus, Kafupi was whisked away in his BMW, and within two minutes the derelict courtroom was again deserted. I went over to the garage to collect my bicycle. Gone! My sturdy Raleigh Roadster. Forty-two years together in Zambia, and now gone. I went back to the lawnmower, sat down and wept.

Then suddenly, screaming into the yard came a white landcruiser, and out jumped a police inspector and four armed paramilitary. 'Spectator Kalaki, you have been found in possession of a lawnmower suspected to be stolen, and stealing a motor vehicle is a non-bailable offence!'

So saying, they picked me up and threw me into the back of the landcruiser and drove off at high speed. 'This is what you get,' cackled the Inspector, 'for encouraging us to do our duty.'

Round and round we went, round the High Court roundabout at a ferocious speed. 'Where are you taking me?' I shouted.

'We don't know,' laughed the Inspector. 'We're waiting for further instructions!'

19th February 2004

Chapter 2
Kings and Things

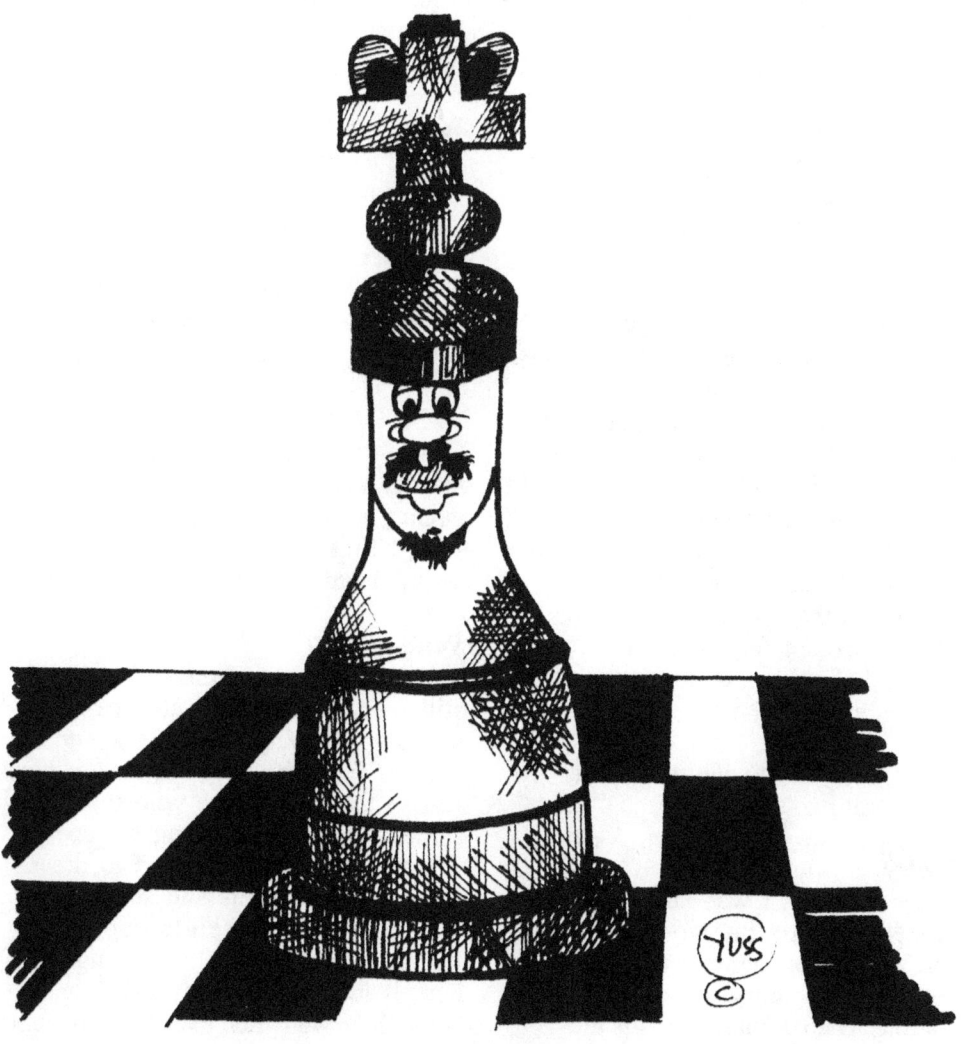

2.1 Kanono's Diary

Thursday

Things are much better here, *Dear Diary,* now that I finally got up the courage to chase the Queen.

How I am enjoying life, all alone with my own dear self, just listening to my own golden voice, with nobody to contradict me. How I enjoy my own excellent company. How I cackle at my own witty remarks! Of all my admirers, I am the one who appreciates me most! Oh my lovely King Kanono, how lucky are my people that God gave them such a prophet, such a Moses, such a political engineer and such a divine dribbler. *Dear Diary,* everyday I humbly congratulate God for making such an excellent choice.

I must divorce her, to make sure she doesn't come back. No wonder the country fell into such a state, with her bossing me around. She was the one who insisted on me declaring a Christian Nation. I only found out afterwards that the Church forbids divorce, except for archbishops. Maybe I should now declare myself an archbishop, in order to divorce her.

Ha ha, I have such a brilliant mind, I am so full of ideas!

Friday

Dear Diary, I was having a peaceful smoke this morning when I had another brilliant idea. I shall declare the country to be a Muslim Nation. Then I shall ring up the Queen on my lovely little gold cell phone, and say *I divorce you* three times. But first I must speak to the unspeakable little Villain Malambo, and tell him to have another fiddle with the Constitution. Then I shall inform my loyal representatives in Parliament to convert to Islam or return their Pajeros.

Saturday

I must have smoked too much yesterday, I had quite forgotten that I'd fired Villain Malambo and abolished Parliament. Now that I've fired the lot, there's nobody to talk to except you, *Dear Diary.* Even the cobra has slithered out under the door.

So today I issued the Executive Order granting myself a divorce. How marvellous to follow the rule of law, when you are the law! Power is sweet! Free again! A young bachelor again! I have recovered my virginity!

Sunday

I hadn't realised the Queen was still so popular. There are crowds at the gate shouting *Bring back our Queen! Fire the King!* Little do they realise that it was she who made such a mess of things, bossing me around. She was the one who used to dress me up in flash suits and shades, making me look like a cheap gangster! Very crafty at making herself look good at my expense. Now they want her back and me out!

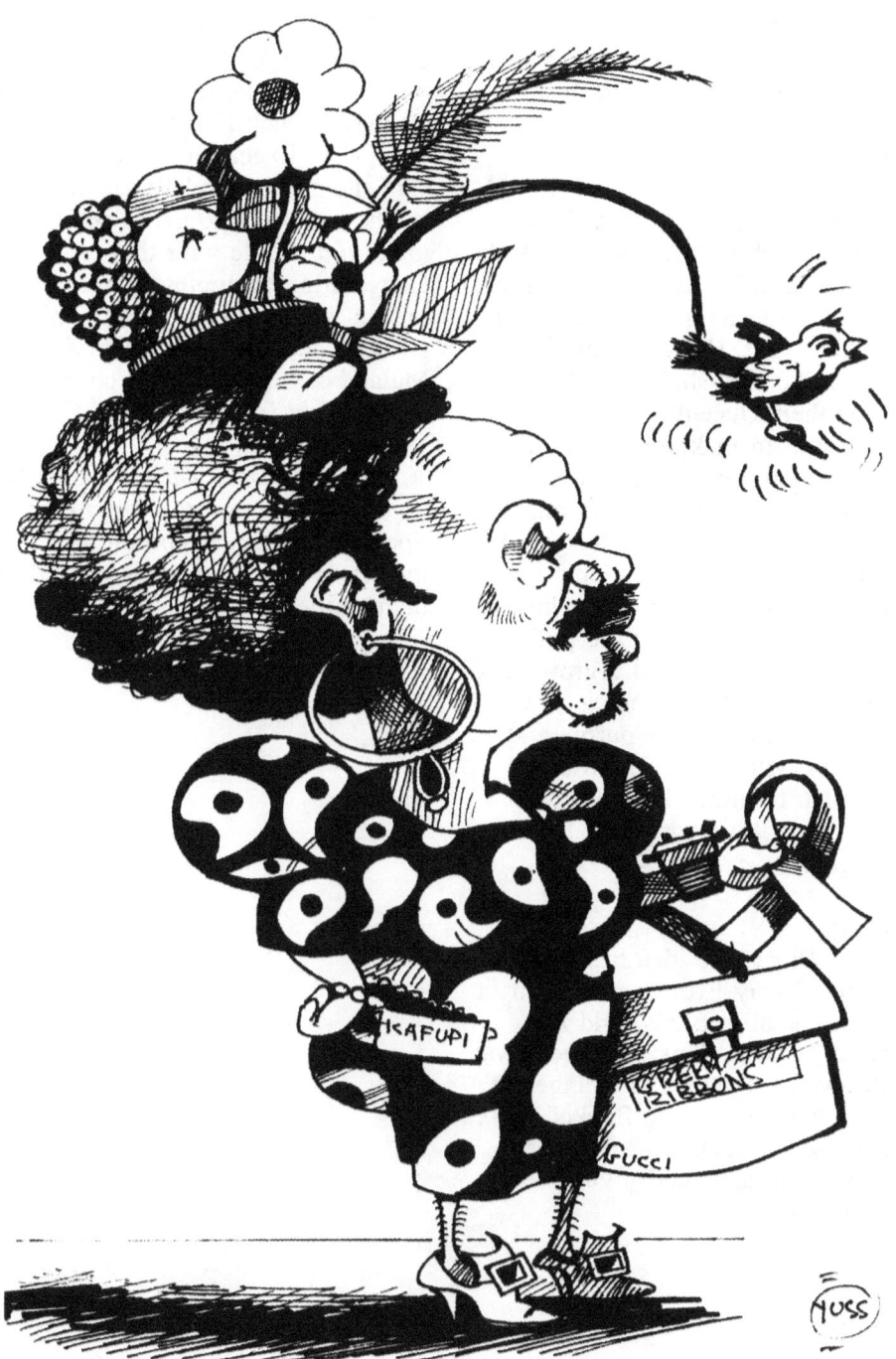

Dear Diary, what can I do?

How did a clever fellow like me get into an awful mess like this?

Monday

Dear Diary, I'm not finished yet! I've had a great idea! Little do they realise that behind these squinty little eyes there is a brilliant political mind. Democracy means giving the people what they want. If they want the Queen back, they shall have her! I shall be their Queen!

I have been making the tea and doing the cooking. I have learnt how to walk in her high heels, so much larger than mine. I am really growing into the role. Not many people realise I am an ingenious engineer, who can change my shape to suit the political environment. I have really grown and developed to fit the demands of the job. When I put on her purple and gold dress with the green stripes, I just couldn't believe how beautiful I was. I fell in love with myself all over again.

Tuesday

Dear Diary, the idea has worked perfectly. Today I drove into town in my gold metallic BMW, and had lunch at Nandos. This time there was no throwing of stones or oranges or rotten tomatoes. People flocked to see their Queen. I spent all afternoon signing autographs and giving out green ribbons.

The next step is simple. I shall choose some dull clod of a man to marry, and make him my King Cabbage. Once I've shown him how to sign an Executive Order, he can sign them everyday! I shall rule him as she used to rule me! Then I shall make him fiddle with the Constitution, changing it to say that only a woman can be king! This time I shan't need any help from Villain Malambo. Instead I shall count on full support from the NGOCC and Women's Lobby!

But now, *Dear Diary*, I must hide you away. Tomorrow morning Spectator Kalaki is coming to interview me. If he reads this, all my plans will come to nothing.

4th October 2001

2.2 Haunted House

Wednesday

Dear Diary, today we moved into our marvellous new home, now that Kabeji has got the top job. The previous tenant, Wabufi Kafupi, was in tears as he handed over. He had kept the house marvellously, but was refused renewal of contract after being caught eating the peacocks and impala.

'Please,' said Kafupi, as we said goodbye, 'don't change anything. Leave it as it is. Even the pictures on the wall.'

Thursday

Kabeji slept like a log last night, after I'd given him his pills. But I just couldn't get comfortable on that mattress. The springs are all finished. 'What was he doing on it?' I asked Kabeji at breakfast, 'to get it in such a state?'

'I'm told he never slept much,' he replied. 'Often he would spend the whole night wrestling with weighty problems.'

'That reminds me,' I said. 'We've got to discuss your acceptance speech. Have a look through this draft, my dear, while you're swallowing your pills. We need a strong message of reconciliation, all work together for the sake of the nation, that sort of thing.'

With a little encouragement from me, he made a first attempt to read it out loud. 'My intention is to appoint some of my opponents to my new team...', he began.

Then he stopped, looked up and seemed to go into a trance. Finally he shouted at me *'But if they oppose me, that is treason, they'll be arrested, found guilty and sentenced to death!'*

I wiped his brow with a white embroidered linen serviette, and got him to lie down on the sofa. 'Don't upset yourself, my dear,' I said gently, as I gave him his medicine. 'We'll have another try tomorrow.'

Friday

Dear Diary, I'm worried that this job may be too much for my husband. At breakfast he did manage to read the second sentence quite nicely. All about the members of his team being people of integrity and honesty, and above reproach, who will put the national interest above personal interest.

But having said this in a calm, magisterial and convincing voice, my husband put down the paper, and looked vacantly into the far distance. Then his face twisted into an ugly sneer, which strangely mirrored the picture of Kafupi hanging on the wall.

'However,' he snarled, clumsily spilling his tea all over the nicely printed speech, *'it is also important that I repay my personal debt to my closest associates. These are the liars, dealers and crooks who gladly and willingly besmirched their reputations in order to devise the various dirty*

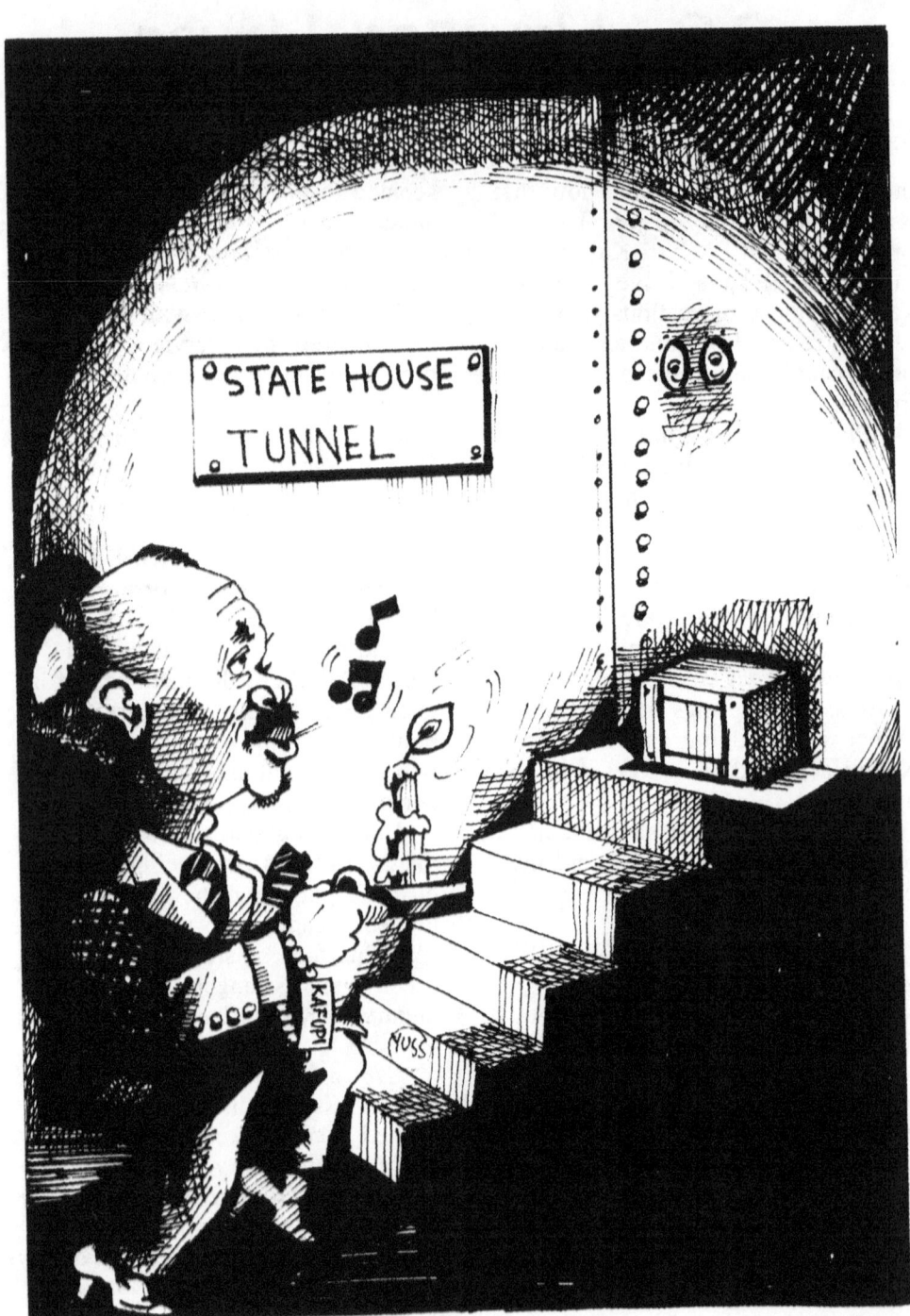

tricks that put me into this high office.'

'Darling,' I said, holding his hand and trying to calm him, 'it would be better if you could just stick to the official text. We are aiming for something calm, diplomatic, reassuring, and statesmanlike. Under no circumstances should you allow yourself to say what is actually on your mind.'

Saturday

I tried again with Kabeji at breakfast, but he was still in a terrible fit, as if he'd been tormented all night by one of the springs in Kafupi's mattress. I got him to read another sentence, saying 'All leaders must be humble and accept criticism, and work amicably with our co-operating partners.'

But he fell onto the floor in a furious rage, shouting, *'I'm not having these donors criticizing our election, or asking what has happened to their funding. What are they doing here anyway?'*

And something very creepy, Dear Diary. He seemed to be looking up at the picture of Kafupi. And when I glanced up at it, I thought I saw the eyes move! Oh My God, am I living in a haunted house?

I was shaking with fear as I gave him some more pills, and laid him down quietly on the sofa.

Sunday

This morning I got up early to make breakfast, and discovered something really ghoulish and goose-pimply about this house. I found the Kafupi picture with empty holes where the eyes should be! But it had eyes yesterday! I got a torch, stood on a chair, and looked inside. A tunnel! I knew it! Kafupi is still here! He's in the tunnels! Casting an evil spell on my husband!

So I arranged breakfast on the patio, away from the evil eye. And do you know, *Dear Diary,* Kabeji read the speech perfectly! No problems at all! Every successful man has a little woman right behind him!

Monday

Today is Kabeji's big day before the cameras. So I buttoned up his shirt properly, straightened his tie, gave him a double dose of pills, and sent him on his way.

Oh Kabeji, your dear wife and the whole nation has so much hope invested in you! Please don't disappoint us!

10th January 2002

2.3 Unity

'TURN on the TV,' said Sara, 'our Great Leader is supposed to be addressing the nation to explain his latest ideas on how we should be governed.'

'How lucky we are,' I sighed, 'that we do not have to trouble ourselves with political problems, but only to put our trust in Him.'

'We must thank the Constitution,' said Sara, 'that conferred upon him the wisdom to decide everything on our behalf.'

A large face filled the screen, as an angry mouth threatened the microphone, and bulbous eyes protruded into the sitting room. Our small grandson immediately burst into a fit of screaming, and ran to hide behind the sofa.

I followed him on all fours. 'Fee fie foh fum!' I growled, 'I smell the blood of a plunderer!'

'Don't torment the poor little fellow,' Sara protested. 'Kupela, take Kondwani outside to play on the swing. This programme is for adults only.'

'The past year has been particularly difficult for this great country,' began the Great Leader. 'There has been too much competition and division amongst ourselves. We need to work together in unity and harmony if we are to solve the great problems this country is facing.'

'The famine?' I wondered.

'He means,' said Sara, 'the problems of minority government.'

'It is these divisions between parties,' continued the Great Leader, 'which have caused so much corruption. When ministers are under scrutiny from the opposition, and might be ousted at any time, they are tempted to steal massively during their short time of opportunity. But if government is shared amongst all parties, we can maintain job security, and share the cake fairly.'

'But surely,' I objected, 'MMD is supposed to believe in competition between parties, as the basis of democracy.'

'Only if they have the majority,' laughed Sara.

'Therefore,' said the Great Leader, 'by virtue of the powers given to me under the Constitution, I shall be appointing ministers from all opposition parties.'

'So they can oppose him from within his own government?' I wondered.

'So they can be bought off,' laughed Sara. 'Anyway, he doesn't have much choice. Half of his party are in jail for theft, and the other half are in court for stealing the last election.'

The camera now moved back to show more of the Great Leader. 'His hair has gone all white!' Sara exclaimed. 'He's even going bald!'

'The worries of high office can cause premature ageing,' I explained.

'Just as there has been wasteful

division in parliament,' declared the Great Leader, 'so there has been destructive competition in the economy. With immediate effect I am amalgamating all banks together under one state bank, to be known as Zambank, with myself as Chairperson.'

At this the audience began to chant, remembering the good old days.

'One Zambia, One Bank,
That Bank, Zambank.'

The camera again moved further back, to show the Great Leader standing in front of his microphone, mopping his face with a white handkerchief.

'Its Mulungushi Hall!' I exclaimed. 'I recognise the lack of ventilation!'

'He's wearing a safari suit and a spotted cravat!'

'Oh My God!' I cried. 'He's becoming just like Old Munshumfwa!'

'And another thing!' the Great Leader snapped at the microphone, 'Why have we got so many football teams, all competing against each other?'

'That's very like Old Munshumfwa!' laughed Sara. 'If he couldn't understand anything, he abolished it immediately! It made the world so much easier to understand!'

'Henceforth,' declared the Great Leader, 'all football teams will be amalgamated into one National Team to be known as Chipolopolo, with myself as Chairman. With only one team, all players will run in the same direction, and goals will therefore become plentiful.'

The camera now moved even further back, to show the audience of men all dressed in safari suits and spotted cravats, standing to salute the Great Leader, and chanting:

One team, one direction,
One direction, one leader,
That leader, Munshumfwa!

'It is Munshumfwa!' shouted Sara. 'He's back!'

'Are you sure?' I said. 'Maybe Mwanamwanamwana is slowly turning into Munshumfwa. All leaders start off being quite reasonable and democratic, but finish up being Munshumfwa.'

'With immediate effect,' declared the Great Leader, 'the Movement for Multiparty Democracy becomes the Movement for Mending Divisions. All members of parliament automatically become members of this new party of national unity. These changes will entail amendments to the Constitution, which will be passed unanimously by parliament first thing tomorrow morning.

'Therefore, I now begin with my list of new appointments. Firstly, I must begin by paying tribute to my young friend Mwanamwanamwana. It is some years since I appointed him State Council, and he has done a commendable job. I am therefore promoting him to be Chairperson of the new National Aids Foundation.'

'Quite right,' laughed Sara. 'It needed a younger man.'

2.4 The Palace

THE guard saluted as I cycled in through the huge front gate, then freewheeled down the long drive, round the flowerbed, and into the great portico. I was propping my bike up against one of the huge pillars when the heavy mukwa door swung slowly open, revealing the massive frame of my old friend Morleen.

'Kalaki!' she laughed, coming out to give me a hug, 'Can't you afford a car?'

'Certainly not,' I said. 'And to be found with a car that you obviously can't afford is a non-bailable offence.'

'This place is very grand,' I said, looking around, as we settled down into the white leather sofa. 'More like a palace. Are you happy here?'

'That's why I asked you round for a cup of tea,' she said. 'This damned palace is becoming a nightmare, and its driving my poor dear husband out of his mind!'

'Poor man, how you've stuck by him! Where is he this afternoon?'

As she spoke there was a shuddering rumbling sound from the heavens, and a piece of plaster fell from the ceiling. 'My God!' I said, standing up. 'An earthquake! Let me go and move my bicycle!'

'Don't be silly,' she laughed. 'That's my Revvy snoring upstairs. I've just given him his pills. Don't worry,' she said, putting her arm round me, 'we're quite safe down here.'

'You know,' I said, giving her a little squeeze, 'I've never understood why you married him!'

'Even me, I sometimes wonder,' she said. 'He's got worse since the accident.'

'What, the car accident?'

'No, the accident of being given this house. It has preyed on his mind, the guilt of getting it by accident, and knowing he didn't deserve it.'

'How did that happen?'

'When the previous owner, a man called Kafupi, had to get out quick.'

'So what made him give it to Revvy?'

'Kafupi had fallen out with all his friends and relatives. Just to spite them, he gave everything to Revvy. So now there's an endless case in court, trying to prove that Revvy is not the rightful owner.'

'Found with a palace suspected to be stolen! And Revvy hasn't even been taken into custody! Surely, stealing a palace is more serious than stealing a motor car!'

'Apparently not,' laughed Morleen. 'If you're charged with stealing a palace, you can even continue to stay in it! Even stealing a bicycle is more serious, because the police will confiscate the bicycle until the case is determined. By the way, where did your bicycle come from?'

'I was given it,' I sniffed, 'by a satisfied customer.'

'Oooh,' she giggled. 'If she'd been more satisfied, she could have given you a motor car!'

'You know,' I said, 'I think Revvy is a lucky man, living here with you. Why can't he just enjoy it while it lasts?'

'Its not just the guilt,' she said. 'You see, living in this palace has had a strange effect on him. If you put a man in a kraal, he begins to behave like a bull. But if you put him in a palace, he begins to behave like a king! Taking charge of everything! Pretending to know everything!'

'All men are like that!' I said. 'Every husband thinks he's the head of the household! A little king! But you're the wife, so its your job to keep him under control!'

'But in a palace, who can control the king? He thinks his powers come from God! Do you know he kicked out all the servants from their quarters, and put in his poor relatives from Chibombo. Now the servants are demanding his arrest for stealing their houses and their housing allowances. And Revvy is demanding their arrest for holding illegal meetings and not bowing when he walks past. He's got everybody in a rage!'

Just then we heard a dull *thud thud*, and a clumsy dishevelled figure came slowly and heavily down the stairs. His vast belly protruded from his crumpled jacket, which he was wearing back to front, and his unlaced boots were on the wrong feet. He marched past without seeing us, his hands outstretched in front of him, bellowing loudly...

'Where are my spectacles? How can I find my spectacles without my spectacles? How can I lead my people without my spectacles?'

So saying, he continued blindly out onto the veranda, tripped over the edge, and fell face first on the gravel drive. We rushed out to help him.

'Leave me alone!' He roared. 'I'm examining this gravel! I'm having the Chief Gardener arrested for stealing the stones!'

'What can I do with him?' Morleen pleaded, turning to me.

'It's a wife's duty,' I said gravely, 'to protect society from her husband. Delusions of kingship are extremely dangerous, and it is most important that you confine him within these walls.'

'Yes,' she said, her eyes glinting, 'then I can be Queen!'

14th August 2003

2.5 The Red Carpet

THE TV picture showed a right royal scene, fit to put before a King. The red carpet had already been laid as the plane taxied to a halt. Then the steps were put in place, and the door swung open. The crowd waited for a first glimpse of their returning King.

'We'd be lost without TVZ,' said Sara, 'to show us how our leaders squander our money.'

A cheer came up from the crowd as the King appeared in the doorway, an ungainly figure, looking more like a sack of mealie-meal dressed up in a suit. Below him, at the foot of the steps there knelt a bald and podgy little fellow, clutching a bouquet of flowers to give to his master.

'See how the greasy Mumbo Jumbo fawns and grovels,' I said.

'It's the same with all of them,' Sara laughed. 'They're very humble when they look up, and very pompous when they look down.'

The King was so delighted to see the size of the crowd that money can buy that he began to dance down the steps to the tune of the welcoming band. But unfortunately his shoes, not being entirely obedient to the wishes of the king, had attached themselves to the wrong feet. Consequently they became entangled half way down, causing the royal personage to lurch forward, and land head first into the flabby fat cushion of Mumbo Jumbo.

'Hurray!' laughed Sara. 'That's the first time Mumbo Jumbo has made himself useful. Maybe the Lord put him on Earth for a purpose after all!'

As all his ministers rushed forward to help, the King rose slowly and unsteadily to his feet. His face was as black as thunder, his eyes wild with rage, his spectacles upside down, as he desperately looked for his left arm, which had disappeared somewhere inside his jacket. At this point a TV reporter thrust a microphone into his face...

'Your Excellency, what sort of landing did you have? Are you pleased to be back?'

The King snarled angrily at the microphone, as if to bite it off. 'This demonstrates what is wrong with this country! In every country I visit I find law and order, and everything done properly, according to due process. But in this country,' he growled, his bulbous red eyes bulging, 'there is nothing but confusion! That is why I launched my War on Confusion. I leave you for just one week, only to come back and find things even worse! Everything is falling upside down again! You see how it takes me and all my ministers to put things the right way up!'

'And can you tell us something about your trip, Your Excellency?'

'I attended the African Development Conference in eh, in eh, in Togo...' An aide approached and whispered in the King's ear, as the King paused and frowned.

'... in Tokyo,' the King continued,

'where the donors agreed to give me another $20 million to assist me in flying round the world, to fight my War on Confusion. Only by looking at law and order in other countries shall I know how to get rid of confusion here.'

'Right now,' said the reporter, 'There's a lot of confusion over the acquittal of the plunderers. What do you say about that? Are we making progress?'

'Let us not, eh, um, er, ah, measury, ah, measure success by the number of convictions.'

'Then shall we measure success by the number of acquittals?'

'Er, errum, you are, ah, I mean this is, er, more a matter of confusion than corruption. The problem in this case was not corruption but confusion. The plunderers were accused of stealing motor cars, but subsequently the defence managed to prove that the vehicles were in fact motor boats and motor cycles, throwing the whole case into confusion.'

'Perhaps the prosecution was corrupted?'

'No, they are just confused villagers who didn't realize that a vehicle without four wheels couldn't be a motor car...'

But as he began walking he tripped over Mumbo Jumbo, who had been licking his boots. His fall, together with a gust of wind, encouraged the undisciplined carpet to begin rolling itself up. All the way to the King's waiting limousine! With the King still trapped inside!

'Usually these interviews end in confusion,' said Sara. 'But this one has been wrapped up nicely!'

'Roll him back,' commanded the Minister for Red Carpets, 'it's the only way to get him out!'

So the carpet was unrolled all the way back to the foot of the steps. Then out staggered the King, even more dishevelled than before. Seeing the steps, up he ran, standing in the doorway, and waving to the crowd!

'Goodbye!' he shouted. 'I'm off to Rio de Janeiro to sign the UN Convention Against Confusion!'

9th October 2003

2.6   Indaba Maningi

IT was Saturday morning outside the People's Palace as the cavalcade of cars and outriders came down the long drive of the People's Park. Then out of a huge limousine wobbled the Wobbly King, his spectacles wobbling on his nose, and his crown wobbling on his wobbly head.

The Secretary to King Wobble, Mr Lazy Mfoola, stepped forward to welcome the King, falling to his knees and grasping both the king's hands, in a gesture of nauseating grovel which enormously pleased the King.

'You ah, you ah, you can ah arise, Mr Mfoola,' said King Wobble with a grand sweep of his arm which swept away Mfoola's spectacles. 'Ar, ar, arise and show me round this Great Indaba!'

'The Wobbly Secretary rose to his feet. 'Thank you, Your Highness. We have invited representatives from every organisation in the country.'

'And ah, whatah, what are they supposed to discuss?'

'That's for them to decide,' chuckled the Secretary. 'We have organisations with opposite opinions on every subject, so although it started quite peacefully, we expect a really huge Indaba by the final day. We even have the Mobile Unit on standby.'

'Whatis er, what is happening over there?' asked the King, pointing his wobbly arm towards some men with rifles prowling stealthily through the distant bushes.

'That's the Safari Hunters Association,' explained the Wobbly Secretary. 'We invited them to shoot the impala, to provide food for lunch.'

'Buttoo, buttoo, but who are those other men, who seem to be hunting the hunters?'

'We also invited the Zambia Wildlife Authority to check if the hunters have licences.'

'But who's driving behind in the landrover?'

'We also invited the Anti-Corruption Commission, to see if ZAWA pockets the fines they collect from the hunters! Just wait until the next impala gets shot, then there's going to be a very big Indaba indeed!'

Now the Wobbly Secretary led the King over to the other side of the park, where horses and riders were galloping up and down at a furious pace. 'Here,' said the Wobbly Secretary, 'we have the Polo Club. They say if we put them in charge of implementing economic policy, everything will move at a gallop!'

'Butwe, um, but we don't have an economic policy.'

'Of course not, Your Majesty. You know that and I know that, but the Polo Club doesn't know that.'

'Hairdo, hairdo, I mean how do, eh, how do they get their horses to gallop so fast?'

'We also invited the Darts Club,

who are throwing their darts from behind those bushes. When the Polo Club finds out, we should have a really big Indaba!'

'It kudu, it kudu cause a great disaster!'

'We've invited the Disaster Management Department to take charge of all the logistics.'

'And what is thatee glate clowd over there?'

'Those are all the representatives from the teachers unions, civil service unions and pensioners. They've gone into alliance with the different miners' associations to dig under the Old Museum, where it is rumoured that plundered resources have been buried.'

'They're all working together,' shouted the King. 'This could be an anti-government plot!'

'But if they find anything,' sniggered the Wobbly Secretary, 'there's going to be the most enormous Indaba!'

'Ivum, ivum, rottenee forgottenee,' said King Wobbly, as he scratched his head and frowned. 'Why are we doing all this? Is it just to cause trouble, and confuse the opposition?'

'You must remember, Your Most Memorable Majesty,' said the Wobbly Secretary, bowing low. 'It was your most memorable idea. Its part of the War on Corruption. All the most famous people in the land are here, playing indaba games. While they're busy, all the Corruption Agencies are also here, examining their cars in the car park. So now we can imprison all your enemies for driving stolen cars!'

'Suppose their cars were not stolen?'

'They'll be in jail for years, trying to prove it!'

And so, after the grand tour of the Great Indaba, the King was escorted back to his limousine. 'You're doing a great job here,' declared the King, as an aide opened the car door.

'Not so fast!' said a uniformed inspector, jumping forward and holding up a piece of paper. 'This car was stolen from Xaviour Shushushu!'

'Don't be silly,' laughed the King, 'it was Xaviour who was accused of stealing it!'

'But the court found it was legally his! So it is you who has stolen it from him!'

As the King was driven away in a police landrover, the Inspector leapt on top of the limousine, waved his hat in the air, and declared 'It is I, the Reverend Mumbo Jumbo, your new King, pursuing the War on Corruption! Bring all your stolen goods to me, and I promise you a place in Heaven!'

'And now,' murmured the Secretary to himself, 'we have Indaba Maningi!'

16th October 2003

Chapter 3
Thoko's Teddy

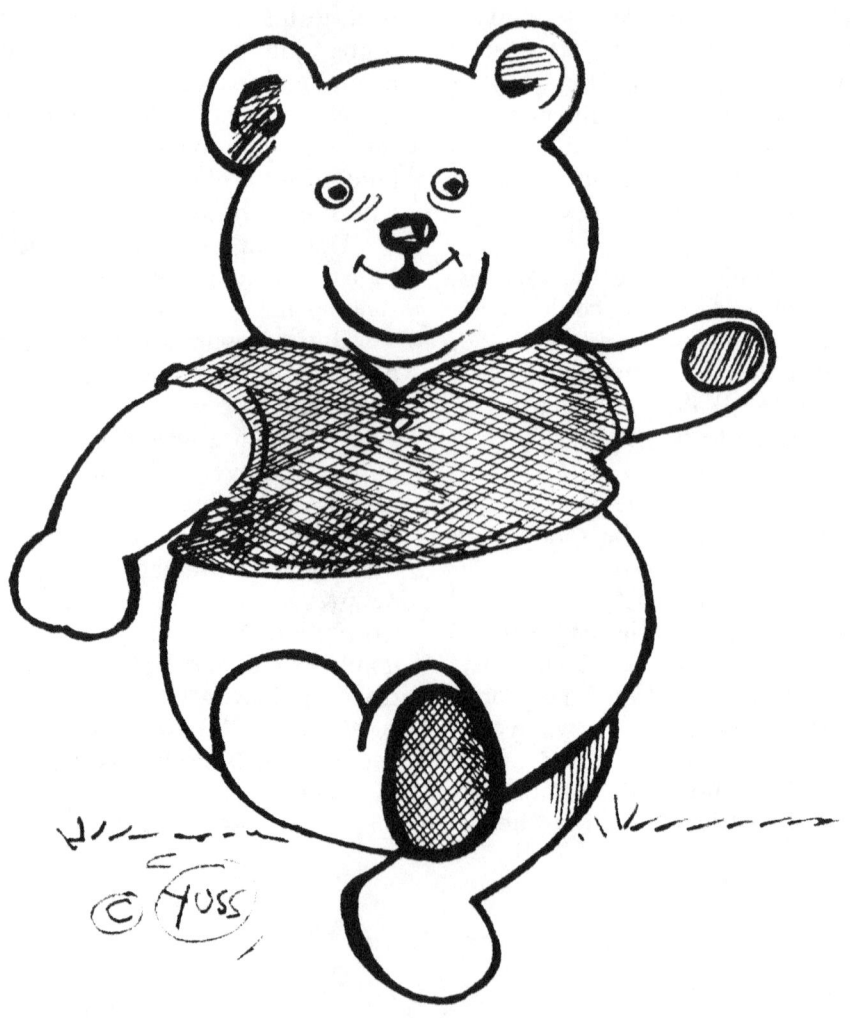

3.1 King Konono

YESTERDAY afternoon my granddaughter Katendi came bouncing in from school.

'Katendi!' I said, bending down to give her a little kiss, 'What did you learn today that you didn't know before?'

'Lots of things you don't know!' scoffed Katendi. 'We learned all about the Sahara. Its just miles and miles of endless sand, and no people at all. Not even old grandpas. We learned all about its history.'

'How does it have a history if it doesn't have people?'

'History, Grandpa, is about the past. A thousand years ago it was the Kingdom of Mukankala, with forests and rivers and millions of people.'

'So what happened?'

'It all went wrong in the time of King Bulili Konono,' explained Katendi. 'Even though he was very small, he was very pompous and greedy.'

'I suppose that's how he became king,' I suggested.

'Not at all,' said Katendi. 'My teacher says kings are appointed by God. But the problem with this king was that he used to take the people's money and never give anything back. The more he had, the more he wanted. He was a kwachamaniac.'

'You mean kleptomaniac.'

'Something like that. He used to keep everything for himself. The more he got, the more he wanted. He just couldn't stop. While the King got richer and richer, the people got poorer and poorer. No medicines in the hospitals and no books in the schools.'

'Just like yours,' I said.

'Yes,' said Katendi. 'That's why we're having to learn about the Sahara. Anyway, one year when the harvest had failed, the people all went to the king to plead for food. Thin and starving, and dressed in rags, they marched on the palace.

'Then out came the king, all dressed in silk and satin, and diamonds and gold, and addressed the people, saying *My heart bleeds to see my people so poor and thin, and I would certainly very much like to help, but unfortunately the government has no money.*

Then a man in the crowd shouted *The King is a thief!* And immediately the police pounced on the man and carted him off to jail.'

'How terrible!' I said. 'Surely he was right! The King was a thief!'

'In those days,' explained Katendi, 'it was a terrible crime to insult the King.'

'But the King was a thief!'

'You don't understand kingship,' said Katendi patiently. 'The King makes the law, and his subjects follow the law. The King is the law. The King cannot be subjected to the law, because he cannot be a subject of himself. According to the rules of kingship, it is impossible for the King to be a thief.'

ARREST LIST
STATE HOUSE
YUSS

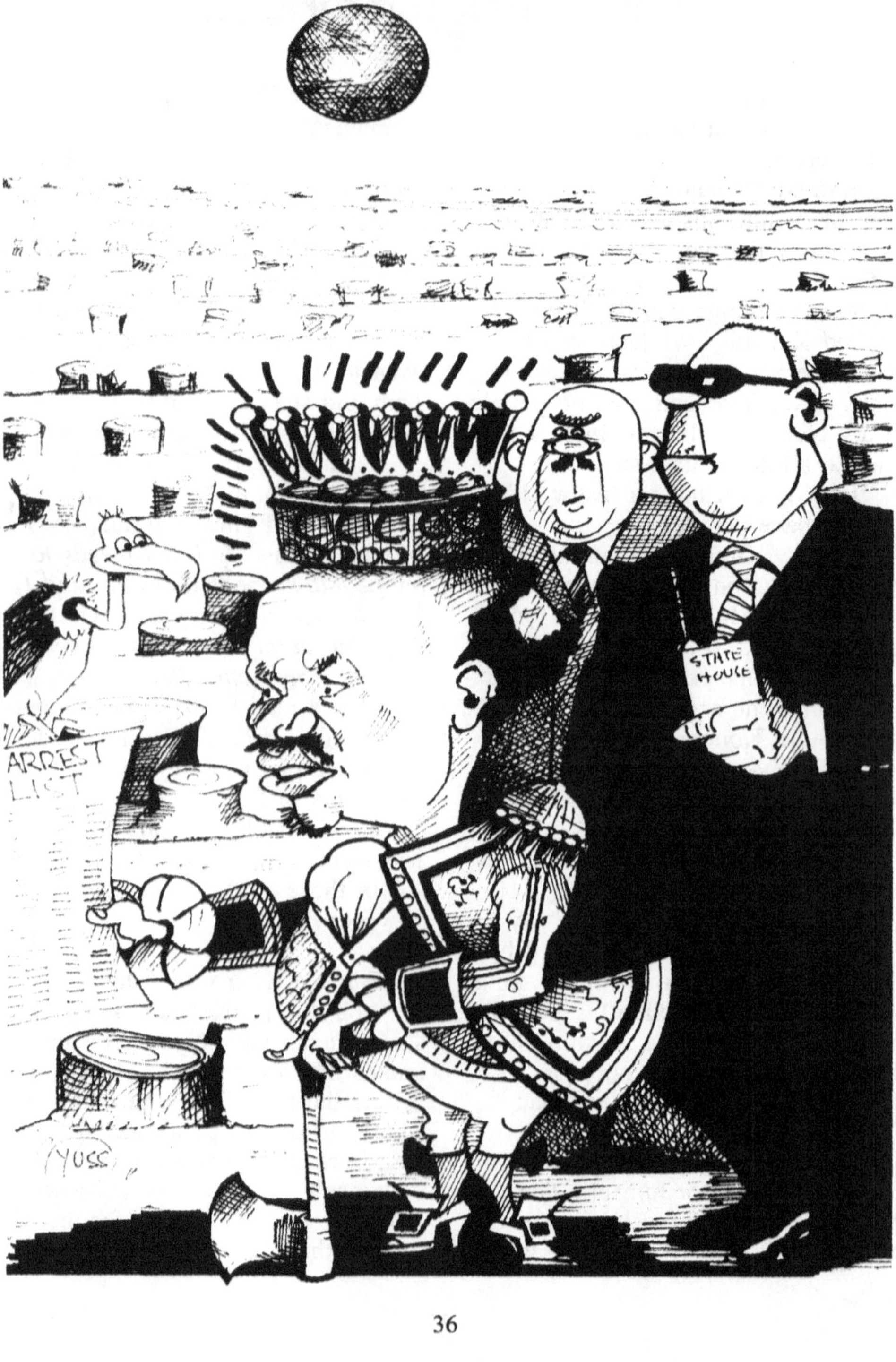

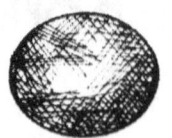

'But was it not those same people, from whom he stole, who appointed him King?'

'Of course not,' laughed Katendi. 'Didn't you do history at school? Kings were appointed by God. To challenge the authority of the king was to challenge the authority of God. How could God make the mistake of appointing a thief? You could be burnt at the stake for such blasphemy!'

'Anyway,' I said, 'what has all this to do with the desert?'

'The trouble was,' said Katendi, 'the people were starving and dying, angry and desperate. The very next day, many other people began to mutter that same treacherous and treasonable phrase that could destroy the state. *The King is a thief!* The King flew into a terrible rage, and sent his police to arrest all the culprits.'

'I suppose things were different in those days,' I admitted. 'But it still seems silly to me if they were arrested for telling the truth!'

'You can't understand this at all, can you Grandpa? Its always telling the truth that gets people in trouble. Only yesterday I was in terrible trouble with Mummy, for telling her that she hadn't washed her face. If they had said that the King was wise, or generous, or tall, or handsome, that wouldn't have got them into trouble. Such lies would have been much appreciated. It's the truth which hurts.'

'So what happened next?'

'People just wouldn't stop saying it. They used to greet each other in the street by saying *The King's a thief.* So before long, everybody except the King and a few policemen were in jail.'

'So that solved the problem?'

'Not at all. Now the King had nobody to steal from, because they were all in jail.'

'So that solved the problem! Now he had to stop stealing!'

'No. Now he stole all the trees. Sold the lot. Within ten years he had turned the whole country into the desert that we now call the Sahara.'

'So what's the moral of this story? That nobody should steal?'

'Certainly not,' said Katendi sternly, 'The moral of the story is that we should respect authority.'

23rd August 2001

3.2 Swallowed

TOWANI brought out some chairs and cushions, and we settled down under the fig tree. We had travelled all the way to Chisamba to see how the next generation was coming along. Our dear daughter had pursued her interest in agriculture even to the extent of marrying a farmer, which I had always thought was taking things a bit too far.

'So where's Yumba?' I asked, looking round.

'He's gone to buy some beer,' said Towani.

'Daddy says you drink too much,' said Thoko.

'Good girl, Thoko!' I laughed. 'Always reporting what Daddy says about poor old Grandpa! How old are you now?'

'Folo,' she said, proudly holding up four fingers.

'You're too small for four,' I scoffed. 'You've not been eating properly.'

'How old are you grandpa?'

'Sickisty,'

'Its you that's not eating properly!' she squealed with laughter. 'Sickisty! You should be as big as this tree by now!'

'I've stopped growing,' I admitted.

'Daddy says you're just drinking beer and swallowing flies. Grandpa, sing me your song about swallowing flies!'

'Stop hitting me with your hat,' I said, 'and I'll begin...

There was an old lady
who swallowed a fly
that tickled and wiggled
and jiggled inside her,
I don't know why
she swallowed a fly,
Perhaps she'll die.'

'Huh,' said Sara, as Thoko clapped her hands in delight, 'Always making fun of women. But its men who are more ridiculous!'

'Good Old Mum,' laughed Towani. 'Always putting Dad in his place. Give us a gender role reversal on swallowing the fly.'

'Hum,' said Sara thoughtfully. 'It would have to go something like this...

There was a Big Man
who swallowed the vote
that rankled and smouldered
and festered inside him.
And all the folk
knew he swallowed the vote,
Perhaps he'll choke!'

'Daddy! Daddy!' Thoko squealed, as Yumba finally arrived with the beer, 'Give Grandpa some beer before he dies!'

'So what's been happening in the local by-election?' I asked, as we poured the beer, 'Do you think they'll vote for Shikashiwa and the Movement for Motor Distribution?'

'He's quite famous,' said Yumba.

'He's been mentioned in both the Gabon Report and the Auditor General's Report.'

'Everybody,' Towani cackled, 'has been mentioned in the Auditor General's Report, except the Auditor General himself.'

'He was also supposed to have been named,' said Sara. 'But he was too modest to mention himself.'

'Then perhaps they'll vote for Lubaluba, of the Up and Down party?'

'I doubt it,' laughed Yumba. 'The voters have already been warned that if they vote against the government then development will come to a standstill.'

'But suppose they still insist on voting for Lubaluba?'

'What goes up must come down. He'll be made a deputy minister, so all his voters will be turned into government supporters!'

'Then development won't come to a standstill after all!'

'Oh yes it will! A deputy minister is given only a small house and an old Volvo, and has no power or influence at all. That's why they were given the warning! He'll be swallowed!'

'Swallowed!' cried Thoko. 'Grandpa, give us some more of your song!'

'There was an old lady
who swallowed a spider,
She swallowed the spider
to catch the fly,
Perhaps she'll die!'

'Come on Mum,' Towani appealed to Sara. 'Give us your version!'

'There was a Big Man
who swallowed the party,
He swallowed the party
to catch the vote,
Perhaps he'll choke!'

'Come on Grandpa,' said Thoko. 'Finish the story! Tell us what happened to the old lady!'

'She swallowed a rat
to catch the spider,
She swallowed the spider
To catch the fly,
I don't know why
she swallowed the fly,
Of course she died!'

'Come on Mum,' said Towani. 'What happened to the Big Man?'

'He swallowed the Parly
to catch the party,
He swallowed the party
to catch the vote,
But all the folk
knew he swallowed the vote,
Of course he choked!'

6th February 2003

3.3 Thoko's Teddy

'GRANDPA!' said Thoko, leaping up and hugging me, and then beginning to pat all my pockets, 'where are my Smarties?'

'Here,' I said, taking a little packet out of my shirt pocket. 'Is it Grandpa you love, or just the Smarties?'

'I love you very much, because you bring me Smarties!'

'And what game are the toys playing this afternoon?'

'We can't play any more!' she said, tears welling into her eyes, as she pointed to all the toys huddled up in one corner. Then she pointed to the opposite corner of the room. 'Uncle Kafupi gave me that big bad Lion yesterday, and now we're all too frightened to play! Why didn't he bring me a nice big Teddy?'

'That reminds me of a story,' I said.

'One upon a time,' said Thoko, helping me to get started, 'there was a big bad Lion, who was King of the Jungle...'

'Exactly,' I said. 'And all the other animals in the forest were very frightened of King Lion, who used to eat up the other animals.'

'The King is supposed to look after his subjects, not eat them up,' said Thoko.

'That's right,' I said. 'Now every evening the animals used to meet at their watering hole, called the Oasis, and complain to each other about Lion, saying he had got too much power...'

'But surely the Lion also had to come to the watering hole, and would have heard their complaints?'

'This King,' I explained, 'never went to the Oasis to mix with the other animals. He always ordered his water to be carried up to the palace in two golden buckets. He knew he wasn't popular, and was scared that all the other animals would gang up on him.'

'But you said he used to eat up the other animals!'

'Yes. But he was very crafty at picking them off, one by one.'

'But wasn't it all these same animals who had elected him King?'

'No. The only ones who voted for him were the lions, crocodiles and hyenas. He got only 29 per cent of the vote.'

'So what was the secret of his great strength?'

'His very strong constitution.'

'What is a constitution, Grandpa?'

'Its how all the different parts fit together. The Lion was always boasting that he had a very strong constitution - with his large powerful stomach serving his enormous muscles, claws and teeth. All the power was his, and nobody would ever topple him!'

'So the animals wanted him to have a different constitution?'

'They said that the constitution should give power to all the animals, not just concentrate all power in the Lion. They said the King should provide food for all the animals to eat, not the King eating all the animals.'

'They wanted a nice big friendly Teddy Bear,' suggested Thoko, 'to organise a Teddy Bear's Picnic, where everybody would stop eating each other, and eat strawberries and cream instead.'

'That's right,' I said, 'A sort of Vegetarian Democracy. So they all met at the Oasis, and decided what to do. They appointed the most talkative animal, a naughty little monkey called Thoko, to put their demands to the Lion King. And Thoko went before the King and said *You must adopt a new constitution. You must stop eating other animals and become a vegetarian. Then your constitution will change. Your claws and fangs will disappear, and your ears will grow bigger so that you can listen to the other animals. Then you will no longer be our Lion. You will be our Teddy Bear, and everybody will love you.*'

'And what did the Lion say?'

"He said *Come closer my dear, so I can digest your ideas!* Then he grabbed the little monkey and swallowed her whole. Then he turned to the other animals and said *When I have digested all this, you shall see what comes out!*'

'Ooh dear,' said Thoko. 'Did all the animals wait patiently to see what came out?'

'No. Thoko's Grandpa, the big hairy Bakolwe Bakalaki was very annoyed. He came along with his big axe and slew the Lion. Then he cut open the belly and pulled out Thoko. Then he took her to the Game Stores, and bought her the biggest ever Teddy Bear. So all the animals were saved, and they all lived happily ever after!'

'Hurray,' laughed Thoko, clapping her hands.

'And what,' I asked, 'is the moral of the story?'

'The moral of that story,' she said solemnly, 'is that if you want to change a lion for a teddy-bear, don't ask permission from the lion.'

'That's right!' I laughed, as we both fell into a fit of laughing, and Thoko threw the Lion out the window.

'Thoko!' said Towani, putting her head round the door, 'Be quiet! You're making too much noise!'

'You also be quiet,' laughed Thoko, 'or I'll change you for Grandpa!'

15th May 2003

3.4　Zoo Story

YESTERDAY morning I was having a late breakfast when I heard a car door bang, then in through the front door strode my grandaughter Thoko, Barbie in one hand and Teddy in the other. 'Mummy's gone to a meeting, so she's dropped me here to look after you. Don't get up, I'll go to the fridge and get myself a Coke.'

'Aren't you supposed to be in school?' I asked, as she came back with a Coke and a packet of Eet Sum Mor.

'You're in a complete muddle as usual, Grandpa,' she laughed, as she stuffed a biscuit into her mouth. 'Katendi is the one who's supposed to go to school, but she doesn't, because the teachers are all on strike. I'm the one who's supposed to go to nursery, except that I don't, because I know everything already. All I have to do is to eat biscuits until I'm big enough to go to Hollywood!'

'The world is a dangerous place,' I said. 'They might eat you!'

'You talk just like Mummy,' she laughed. 'She says you can only get to the top by natural selection.'

'You mean national election.'

'Please listen carefully, Grandpa, I'm talking about natural selection. Only the people who are biggest and greediest and fiercest get to the top. That's why I'm eating all these biscuits, so I don't end up like you, Grandpa!'

'Is that what Mummy says?'

'Yesterday Mummy took me to the zoo at Wonder Mango. We were taken round by one of the elephants, called Nalumango.'

'Are the elephants in charge of the zoo?'

'Of course they are, Grandpa, don't you know anything? As Nalumango explained, being much bigger and stronger, they are in charge of the mangoes, and therefore in charge of everybody.'

'They eat mangoes?'

'Really Grandpa, that's why the place is called Wonder Mango, because it's a mango economy. According to Nalumango it says in the scriptures that in the beginning all animals were the same size. In those days there were big monkeys and small elephants, and all mangoes were shared equally amongst them.'

'Paradise,' I said.

'Nalumango said it was absolute hell, because elephants need much more food so they can grow big and fat, whereas monkeys are quite happy if they're small and thin.'

'So the elephants reorganised things?'

'Structural adjustment,' said Thoko. 'They organised the monkeys to pluck the mangoes from the trees, and the zebras and eland to carry them to the Elephant House.'

'Which soon became the Elephant Palace?'

'Have you heard this story before?' snapped Thoko. 'When each animal brings a hundred mangoes to the Palace its allowed to keep one, since elephants are very generous, and all members of the Rotary Club. So this is how elephants became larger, and all the other animals became smaller.'

'Suppose one of the workers keeps too many mangoes for himself?'

'Culprits are thrown to the lions! Lions are the police force, employed to protect the well fed from the hungry.'

'So which ones are the priests?'

'The vultures. They dispose of all the dead bodies, and carry them up to heaven.'

'And do they do good business?'

'The most profitable business in the whole zoo! The vultures are almost as fat as the elephants and lions. But all the other animals are very thin and sickly.'

'Don't the elephants sometimes have extra mangoes that they can give back to the starving workers?'

'I asked about that. But Nalumango said all the extra mangoes have to be made into mango jam, which is sold to America, where humans have now become as fat as elephants.'

'But why do they have to sell the extra mangoes to America?'

'Mainly because they have to pay back the huge loan that the Americans gave them to build the jam factory. But also because the elephants have bought hundreds of huge Mercedes.'

'Good God!' I exclaimed. 'What for?'

'Really Grandpa!' Thoko laughed, 'it takes four Mercedes to carry just one elephant!'

'But why can't they just stay in Wonder Mango and manage the mango crop?'

'Look,' explained Thoko, 'these are not ordinary animals like you and me. The Chief Elephant has to represent the Zoo at international conferences. When Mummy and I were there we saw a delegation of fifty elephants setting off for a conference in Tanzania.'

'A conference about what?'

'About how to save starving animals in Africa.'

'Weren't other animals angry? Didn't they throw stones as the delegation drove past?'

'Oh no, they cheered and waved!'

'They were really happy?'

'Of course. While the elephants are away they'll have plenty to eat.'

'But surely, one day the little animals will rebel against these monsters!'

'Mummy says that if a single ant climbs up inside an elephant's trunk, it can eat the brains.'

'That could explain everything,' I said. 'It must have already happened!'

4th September 2003

3.5 Up and Down

YESTERDAY afternoon I was sitting on the veranda staring into space, when round the corner came breezing my granddaughter Katendi, swirling school uniform on skinny legs, and bright eyes bursting with mirth. 'Poor Grandpa! This is where I found you sitting last Friday! Are you stuck in the chair!'

'I'm told that your Daddy took you with him to Solwezi last week-end. Tell me all about it.'

'Daddy took me to see the by-election.'

'Which one?'

'At Solwezi game park. There's a place come vacant at the Manda Hill Zoo, so all the animals in Solwezi Game Park are competing for it. The winner is allowed to put his greedy snout in the public trough, and eat free for ever at public expense!'

'Are you sure the by-election is in the Solwezi game park, and not the town?'

'Oh no. Daddy says politics is more suitable for monkeys, hyenas, crocodiles and snakes.'

'So what was it like, in the game park? Parched and bare with starving animals?'

'Good gracious no!' laughed Katendi. 'They have electricity and piped water, green grass and fountains everywhere, with lakes and swimming pools. There are animal clinics, monkey houses in the trees, and a huge crocodile farm.'

'Maybe the place has been sold to South African crocodiles.'

'Maybe the crocodiles actually own the place, but its the elephants who are always bossing everybody around, and imagine they're in charge. Daddy says it's the crafty cheeky monkeys who are busy manipulating all the others.'

'So why is there a by-election? Don't they already have a representative at Manda Hill?'

'In the last election they elected a naughty monkey called Tentemanishiwa, of the Up and Down Party.'

'So what happened to him? Did he die? Overeat and burst? Fall Down and not get Up?'

'He was so pleased to go Up to Manda Hill Zoo, but when he got there he found he had been cast Down. The elephants of the Mighty Mammoth Development party were entirely in charge, and he was just a little monkey in a big zoo. He realised that he would never get any of the big juicy mangoes. Just a few peanuts might be thrown his way if he were lucky.'

'So don't tell me, he refused to be cast Down. The only way to succeed in life is to rise Up after you have been cast Down. So he decided to rise Up by becoming an elephant!'

'Quite right, Grandpa! He went to see the Chief Elephant, the Great Leviathan, who was very clever at imagining he was in charge of everybody. Leviathan offered to swallow him, saying 'I have a belly full of sweet mangoes. Just crawl up my bum and eat them all, then you will get so fat that you can be born again as an elephant.'

'So was he born again as an elephant?'

'Oh yes,' said Katendi, 'After he came back Down, he really rose Up. He's now really fat, just like an elephant. But still rather smelly after his disgusting experience.'

'But can't he still represent the monkeys, now he's on the Up and Up? Because if he risks a by-election, he might go Down!'

'The problem is that the monkeys had voted for a monkey to represent them, not an elephant. So now Tentemanishiwa is standing as the elephant, and Linga Longa is standing as the monkey, promising to linger longer before he changes into an elephant.'

'And did you see the by-election in progress?'

'We saw the Chief Elephant, the Great Leviathan, getting himself into a mammoth rage, shouting at the monkeys and calling them fools. 'Heh heh heh,' he was trumpeting, 'The Up and Down party has got everything upside down. I don't need a monkey to represent you, or to advise me, because the Down cannot advise me who is Up. I need an elephant to represent me and advise you, because it is I who am Up who must advise the Down. So you'd better decide whether you want to come Up, or remain Down!'

'But Katendi, you said the game park is already well Up!'

'That's right, but the Great Leviathan never allows little facts to spoil a big argument. The crafty monkeys have now caused so many by-elections that Solwezi is now the richest game park in the country. All the other game parks have become deserts, while Solwezi gets richer and richer!'

'So now they'll vote for Linga Longa, and have another by-election when he also turns into an elephant!'

'No, they're all voting for Tentemanishiwa, who'll soon turn back into a monkey!'

'What goes Up must come Down!'

'Daddy says there's an old Kaonde saying that *Its difficult to make an elephant out of a monkey, but easy to make a monkey out of an elephant.*'

18th September 2003

3.6 The Plunderer

'GRANDPA,' said Katendi, 'tell us a bedtime story.'

'This is the story of the Plunderer, I began. 'Once upon a time, a long time ago, the Land of Kalaki was infested with lions, who terrorised everybody. But there came a brave young leader who they called the Thunderer, because he thundered around the land on a bicycle, speaking such fiery words that he frightened the lions, who all ran back to England.'

'So Thunderer became King,' said Khoza.

'Exactly,' I said. 'In gratitude the people bought their new King a big aeroplane, since kings shouldn't travel by bicycle. And the King declared that the plane would be like an eagle, flying out with copper and coming back with gold. And so the plane was called the Nkwazi.'

'Did he ever bring back any gold?' asked Katendi.

'Nothing,' I laughed. 'Apart from thundering, the King's only talent was spending. He wasted all the copper money on shopping trips, buying clothes and big motor cars.'

'Why big cars if he'd already got an aeroplane?'

'Because,' I said, 'he used to take a hundred parasites and freeloaders with him, arriving at the airport in a convoy of twenty-four Benzes. Their job was spending the money. That was in addition to their more menial jobs of licking his boots, combing his hair, wiping his nose, and worse.'

'So the poor people remained poor?'

'The people became poorer while the King and his cronies became richer. Then up stood a little Kadoli with beautiful words, saying the Thunderer is no Saviour, he is just a Plunderer. But I am the Orator who will take the wealth of the Plunderer and give fair shares to everybody.'

'So did he become King Kadoli or King Orator?'

'Neither,' I laughed. 'He became known as King Dribbler.'

'Why was that?'

'Because all his fine words were really just useless dribble, which used to continuously dribble out of his mouth and down his chin.'

'So he was a different sort of king?'

'Oh yes,' I laughed. 'He challenged the whole philosophy of the Thunderer!'

'What is philosophy, Grandpa?'

'Philosophy is the lies people tell to stay in power.'

'That's why we listen to you, Grandpa. So how did the Dribbler change philosophy?'

'Instead of flying East to buy Mao suits from China, he now flew West to buy Mafia suits from Manhattan. Because of this challenging change in direction the plane was re-named the Challenger.'

'But which one was the Plunderer?' asked Khoza. 'The

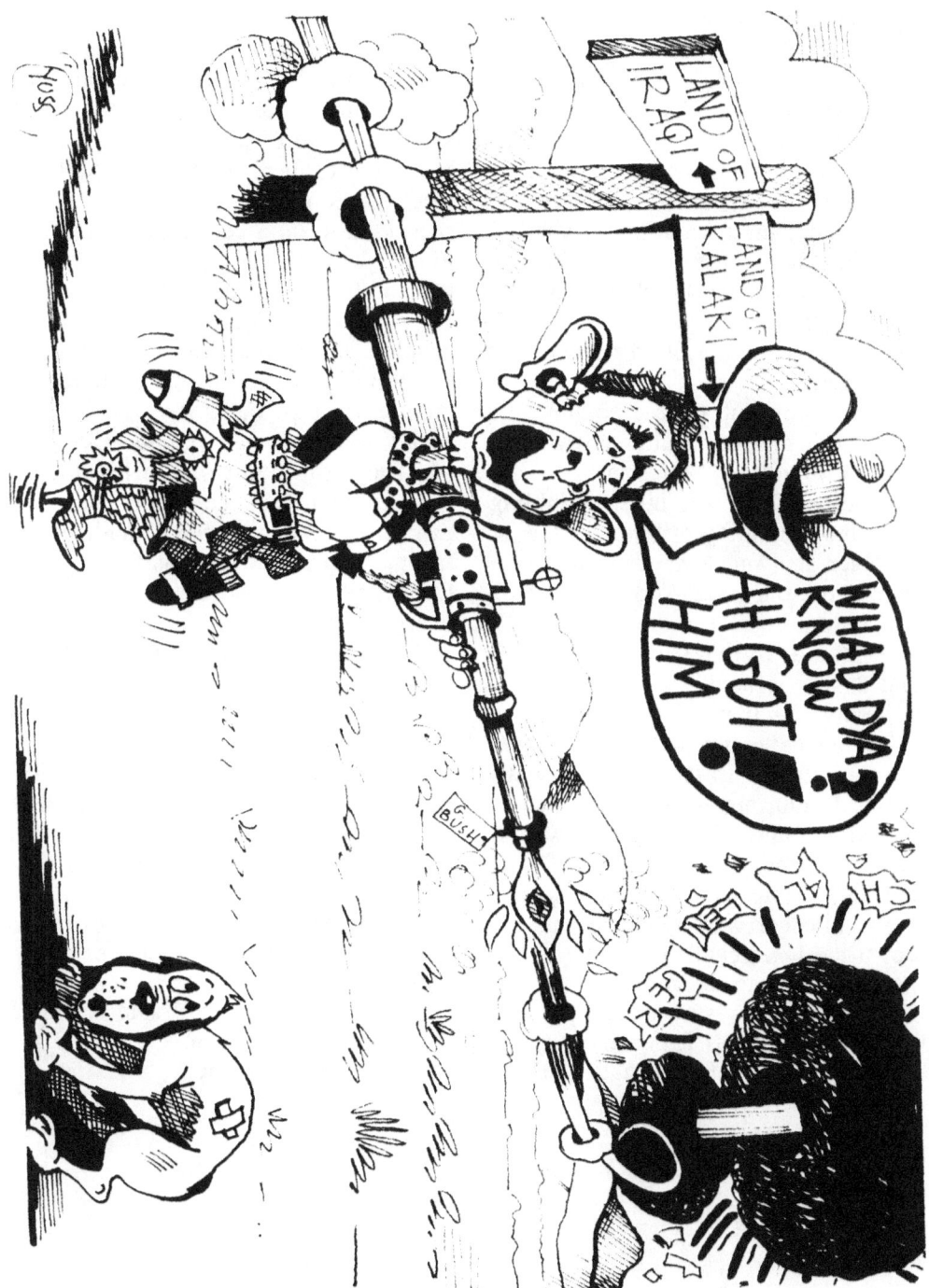

Thunderer or the Dribbler?'

'Which do you think?' I asked.

'Perhaps,' said Katendi, 'It was the plane which was really the problem!'

'The next king,' I continued, 'was called the Stutterer, and he...'

'Why was he called the Stutterer?'

'Because his regime had a very stuttering start, after the Stutterer had blurted out that the Dribbler was really a Plunderer.'

'But perhaps the Stutterer was also a Plunderer?'

'To begin with people couldn't decide whether the Stutterer was really a Plunderer, or just a Blunderer. There was much quibbling from the remaining dribbles of the Dribbler, and much murmuring throughout the land. And the more the murmuring, the more the new King had to fly the Challenger up and down the land.'

'Why was that?'

'The Challenger had to challenge the murmuring. In those days it was illegal to murmur in the presence of the King. Otherwise the police would arrest you for treason under the Public Murmuring Act. So every day the Challenger was flying up and down the land, challenging the people's right to murmur!'

'And did they stop murmuring?'

'No, because as it became worse, so the expenses of the Challenger jet increased tenfold, causing some treasonable muttering in addition to the scurrilous and illegal murmuring. The King had to put a tax on salaula to raise money for fuel, but still the jet needed more, causing the muttering to increase. So then he had to close the university, which was suspected to be a centre of muttering. Finally, as muttering got worse, he had to shut down the civil service. Now the whole country was at a standstill. Only the king's aeroplane could move, as the people muttered quietly amongst themselves, *plunderer, plunderer, plunderer.*'

'They still didn't realise that the Plunderer was not the Stutterer, or even the Dribbler or the Thunderer, but the real Plunderer was the Challenger that was just eating up everything!'

'No. They foolishly imagined that the King was in charge.'

'So they all died?'

'No. One lucky day a confused man called George Bush, who didn't even know the difference between the Land of Kalaki and the Land of Iraqi, sent his missile the wrong way. The Challenger was accidentally blown up. After that nobody wanted to be King, because there wouldn't be any more shopping trips.'

'No more Plunderer!' said Katendi, clapping her hands. 'So everybody lived happily ever after!'

20th March 2003

Chapter 4
Mumbo Jumbo

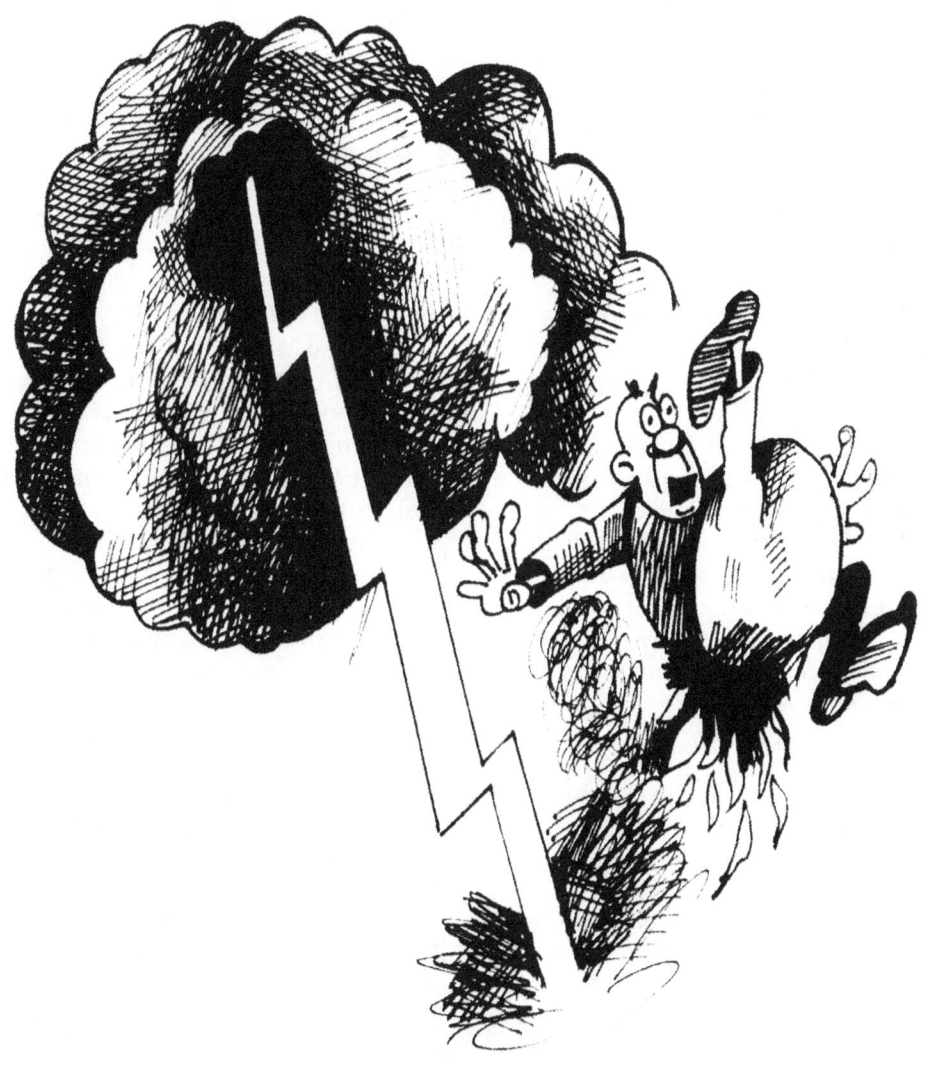

4.1 Never!

'THE Lesson this morning,' shouted the priest, 'is taken from the Gospel according to St Kalaki, Chapter 26, Verses 1-24.'

'Why's he shouting like that?' I whispered to Sara.

'They were all taught to shout at the Bible Shouting School in Kansas,' she explained. 'They shout so you don't fall asleep. This is the Church of Never Mumble, of the Victory Ministries.'

'Victory over sleep?'

'No. Victory over corruption. This Church is very much against corruption!'

'Are some churches in favour of it?' I asked.

'Shush!' said Sara, 'Be quiet and listen to the reading!'

'I've heard it all before,' I sighed. 'Why do they keep reading over and over from the same book?'

'Then Never Mumble sat down with his twelve disciples,' the priest continued, still shouting, and now also jumping up and down with the Gospel in his hand, 'And he said unto them *There is one amongst us, with his hand on this table, who will betray me!*

'And the disciples protested, saying *Betray, Never! We shall find the traitor in our midst, and expel him from the party!*

'But Never spoke unto them again, saying *What I have said is already written, and what is written must come to pass. After the betrayal, you must go out into the world and preach the gospel of the Never Corruption Campaign, according to the Six Commandments of our Manifesto:*

Speak the truth;
Be transparent;
Be accountable
Elect leaders;
Respect the law;
Do not corrupt the Constitution.

'*And now my friends,* said the Lord Never to his disciples, *it is time for me to take my leave, for I hear my Father calling me.*

'And so it was that the disciples were left high and dry, for the Lord was the only one who knew the trick of turning water into wine. And without their usual wine to maintain their conviviality, the disciples began to fall out amongst themselves, accusing each other of betraying the Lord. Florence turned on Peter, saying *Yesterday, as the cock was crowing, I heard you talking to a man and denying that you're a friend of our Lord. You said you never knew him!*

'But Peter answered Florence, saying unto her *I never said I never knew him, I said to him I knew Never.*

'Then Eva turned on Judas Iscariot, saying *You even sold your own sister for thirty pieces of silver, so maybe you even sold our Lord.*

'But Judas answered her, saying *That was my sister's lobola, and she was worth twice as much!*

'And Timothy the Peacemaker tried to calm them, and restore their confidence, saying *I'm sure our Lord can pull off just one more miracle, and avoid the crucifixion.*'

'Florence and Eva?' I whispered to Sara. 'I didn't know there were women amongst the disciples!'

'They all wore long frocks in those days,' she explained. 'It was very difficult to tell the difference.'

'And then Paul,' shouted the priest, 'being one of the more practical amongst the disciples, had the sense to turn on the TV, saying *Verily I say unto you, if he's been betrayed, it'll be on the 10 o'clock news.*'

'I didn't know they had TV in those days,' I whispered to Sara.

'They had everything, until the Catholic Church turned off all the lights, and introduced the Dark Ages.'

'And so it came to pass that the Lord appeared again before the disciples, with his arm round King Herod, saying *The Lord My God has just revealed to me that for the past three years King Herod and myself have been using the same speech writer. This means, unbeknownst to each other, we have been using exactly the same list of Six Commandments on Corruption:*

Speak the truth but protect official secrets;
Be transparent but avoid indecent exposure;
Be accountable but conceal all records;
Elect leaders except for those appointed;
Respect the law or otherwise change it;
Do not corrupt the Constitution except under the Inquiries Act.

'Then Judas Iscariot became sore annoyed, saying unto the others *You see, our Lord Never Mumble is the one who has betrayed us!*

'But Eva answered him, saying *He is our Leader, chosen for us by God. We may betray him, but he cannot betray us. Never! We must follow him wherever he leads, otherwise we shall have betrayed him.*

'And so it came to pass that Eva and the disciples followed their leader into the King's palace, where they were all eaten at the next banquet. And so Eva became our first Christian martyr, St Eva the Trustful.'

'So what is the lesson we learn from this story?' asked the priest, as he closed the Holy Book and leaned towards the congregation. 'We learn from St Eva that we must trust our leaders.'

'Never!' said Sara.

29th May 2003

4.2 Mumbo Jumbo

BISHOP Bling Bling heaved his huge bulk into the pulpit, his gold chains and diamonds glinting in the dazzling shaft of sunlight that God had carefully arranged to shine down on him, while the rest of the congregation remained sitting in the dark.

'What are we doing here?' I whispered to Sara.

'You've become too agnostic,' she said. 'I've brought you here to restore your faith.'

'Huh,' I grunted. 'Their senseless rituals are more likely to restore my faith in rational thought.'

The Bishop laid his gold watch on the lectern, looked over his gold-rimmed spectacles, pushed out his vast belly, and ponderously began to address the congregation. 'We are gathered here today at the Church of the Never Christian Coalition...'

'Never Christian?' I hissed to Sara. 'Are they not Christians?'

'The church was founded by Never Mumbo Jumbo,' Sara patiently explained, 'so they call themselves the Never Christians.'

'If they're Never Christians, they'll never get to Heaven!'

'Can you just keep quiet,' she snapped, 'and listen to what Bishop Bling Bling is blinging.'

'... for it is written in the Gospel according to St Kalaki, Chapter 4,' Bling Bling was rattling on, as religious emotion rattled his gold chains, 'that in the beginning Our Founder grew up as any ordinary young man, very keen to become successful and rich. But he was never willing to do any work, so his friends called him Never. And he constantly bored everybody by talking endless nonsense, so his friends also called him Mumbo Jumbo. And so it came to pass that he became known as Never Mumbo Jumbo.

'And one day his mother Mary said unto him *Son, God in his wisdom has given you soft hands which must not be soiled, a smooth tongue to talk persuasive nonsense, and a great desire to be rich. This is a sign that God has designed you to become a priest.*

'For in those days God never spoke to Never directly, so he had to listen to his mother. And his mother said unto him *You must go to the Land of Big Talk, and learn the evangelical miracle of extracting money from pockets with your tongue.*

'And so in the fullness of time Never Mumbo returned from the Land of Big Talk with his Mumbo more Jumbo than before, with his tongue well oiled, and with a vocabulary even bigger than his head. He was now uniquely qualified to converse directly with the Lord, and to pass on the Lord's latest thoughts to a grateful congregation.

'And so it was that Never Mumba soon established his own Never Christian Coalition, asking his faithful followers to *Praise the Lord and donate generously, so that the Lord*

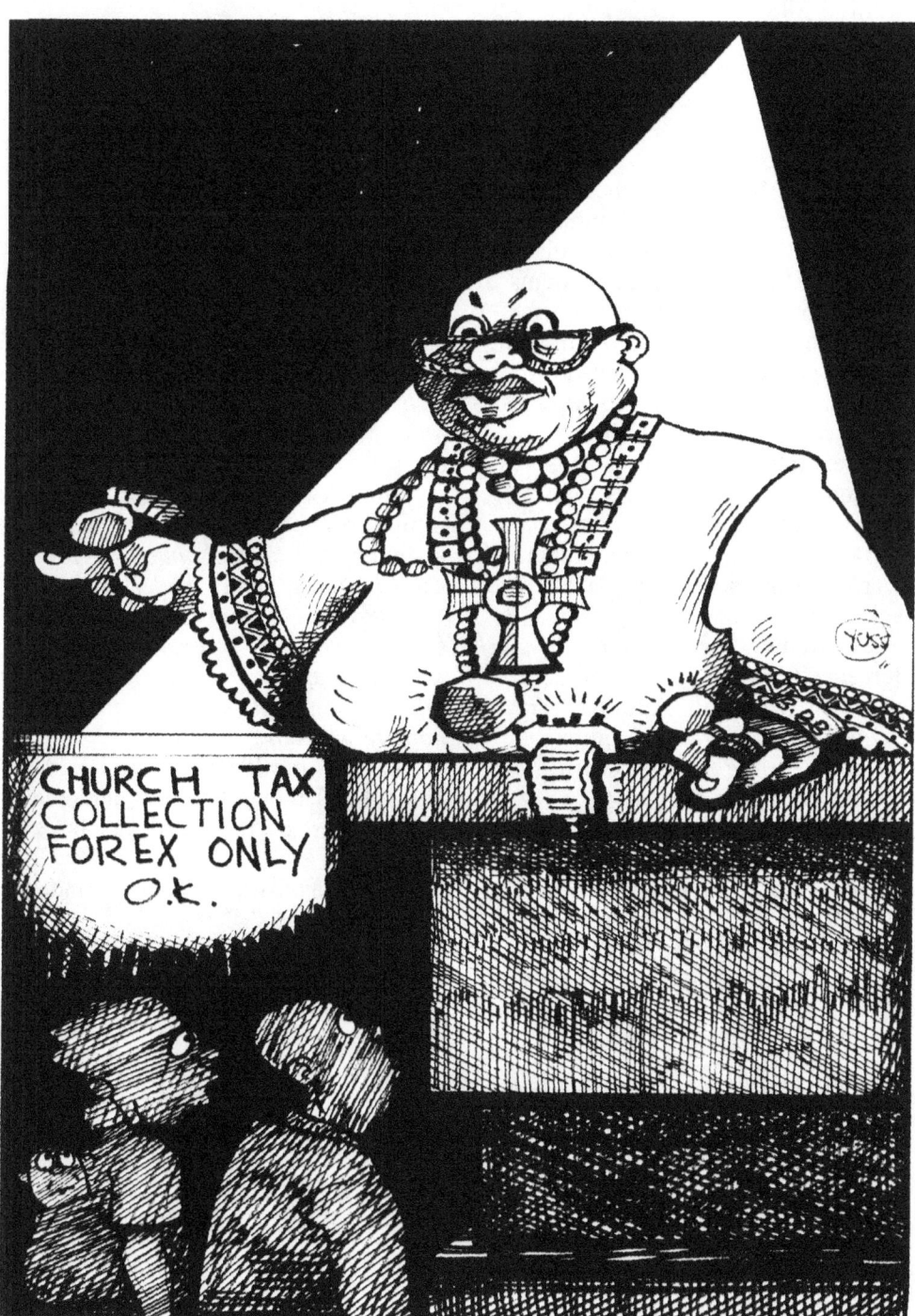

will favour you with His wealth, just as He has favoured me.'

'Hallelujah!' chanted the congregation.

'But as time went on,' continued Bling Bling, 'priests in other churches became sore jealous of Mumbo, who alone could perform the heavenly miracle of hoovering large amounts of money from the pockets of the rich. And so the pharisees, rabbis, mullahs and pickpockets all denounced Mumbo, saying that he was a fraud, who became richer while his followers became poorer.

'And so it came to pass that Mumbo lost his power as his followers lost faith. His congregation shrank and his collection plates came back empty.

'So Mumbo Jumbo drove his Mercedes forty miles into the desert for a chat with God. And the Lord said unto him *If you are hungry, I can give you the power to turn these desert stones into nshima.*

'But Mumbo answered him, saying *Don't trouble yourself, for I have brought a pizza from Debonairs.*

'And the Lord was irritated with his arrogance, saying *If you are thirsty, I can give you the power to turn this desert sand into chibuku.*

'But Mumba answered him, saying *Don't worry, I have champagne in my dashboard cocktail cabinet.*

'Then God took him up onto a high mountain where he could look down on the entire country, saying *I can give you power over all this if only you will prostrate yourself before me. You will be king, and have power to collect taxes, not only from the rich, but even from the poorest of the poor. Much better than any little collection plate!*

'*Now you're talking,* said Mumbo, turning off the car radio and paying attention. *If I am appointed by You, I shall be the greatest leader ever!*

'*That's right,* said God. *With my backing, you will command the greatest respect. You will be able to talk nonsense all the time, and nobody will dare to laugh!*'

'Correct me if I'm wrong,' said Sara, 'but I thought he was tempted in the desert by the Devil, not by God.'

'As an agnostic,' I said, 'I find it hard to tell the difference.'

10th July 2003

4.3 God's Plan

'SPECTATOR Kalaki! How nice to see you again!' he said, as we shook hands, and settled into two comfortable armchairs, his emerald and diamond rings glinting in the morning light. 'What can I do for you this morning?'

'I just hoped you could spare me a few words on your nomination to the House. I saw you being sworn in yesterday. It was a very moving occasion.'

'Very moving indeed!' he sniggered, 'Apparently everybody chose that very moment to go to the toilet! Something must have moved their bowels!'

'Never mind,' I said, putting my hand on his arm to comfort him. 'At least you've made a start. I'm sure you'll be able to move their hearts and minds in due course.'

'Its all in the hands of the Lord!' he said, raising his hands towards the chandelier. 'That's what scares them! They realise that God is now taking charge of this mess! That's why they all ran away!'

'Scared of the Lord?'

'I wouldn't put it quite like that. They've all been brought up in the parliamentary tradition. They think the oath of allegiance means swearing to speak for the people who elected them, and promising to uphold the constitution.'

'And isn't it?'

'Perhaps it is for them!' he laughed, 'Such ordinary mortals, whose bowels are so easily affected by the sight of the Lord's messenger! But for me, the oath of allegiance is my covenant with the Lord.'

So saying he rose from his armchair and picked a red leather bible from his desk, which he waved in the air as he paced around the room, his green velvet suit shaking with religious fervour. 'I am not one of those ordinary mortals who needs to be elected. I have been nominated by the Lord my God to do His will on Earth. I am not here to tell God what the people want, but to tell the people what He requires of them! That is God's Plan! That is what we mean by a Christian Constitution!'

'Come and sit down,' I said soothingly. 'Your cup of tea is getting cold. Tell me the secret of your success.'

'You've already seen it,' he gasped, as he flopped back into his chair, exhausted by his exertions on behalf of the Lord. 'Taking oaths of allegiance. Making covenants with God. I'm enormously convincing. It comes over me like a religious conversion. I even manage to convince myself, such is my faith in the Lord. That's the secret of my success.'

'And when did it all start?'

'At secondary school. One day I went into the headmaster's office, bible in hand, and said *Nominate me as Headboy, and I swear by Almighty God that we shall all pass our Form*

V. Then I went to the boys and said *Each of you donate ten gluders to my Exam Victory Ministry, and I swear by Almighty God that victory will be ours!*'

'And did it work?'

'Oh yes. I became Headboy, and very rich.'

'Yes, but did they all pass?'

'Those were early days in my career, and I was still learning. Unfortunately I was let down by the printer who was supposed to produce the certificates. But I myself managed to pass Religious Education, and was able to afford further studies at Kansas Bible College. That was where I learnt how to use the Good Book even more profitably, in the service of the Lord.'

'Then you came back here?'

'Yes. The Lord nominated me as Director of Visionary Ministries, and I swore a covenant with the Lord that He would give me a vision every Sunday morning at 10 o'clock, and a miracle at 11 o'clock if we were on TV.'

'And so your church prospered?'

'Oh yes, especially after I swore an oath before the congregation that if they would give ten per cent of their salary to the church, the Lord would find them a place in heaven.'

'And did it work?'

'It was a miracle! Even I was surprised. In fact it was far too successful. I soon became very rich, but they all went to heaven. So I was left without a congregation!'

'So you decided to go into politics.'

'Yes. The Lord told me in a vision that what I had done for my congregation, I could now do for the whole country.'

'But you failed miserably at the general election. What went wrong?'

'I was let down terribly by the printer in Kitwe who was supposed to be producing my ballot papers.'

'And now, following your unexpected appointment, all parties are working together on the impeachment of the President! Wouldn't that leave you in charge?'

'That's right. First we unite the country, then I take over! That's God's plan!'

31st July 2003

4.4　Voice of Vice

'ITS past seven,' I said, 'let's turn on the news.'

'While its still free,' laughed Sara. 'Next month we shall be paying K3,000 for the privilege of having our intelligence insulted.'

'Then why do we turn it on every night?' I asked. 'Is it masochism on our part, that we volunteer for such degrading punishment?'

'We should think of it as our daily test of moral integrity and independence,' suggested Sara. 'To test our ability to maintain our belief in human nature, despite the un-edifying spectacle of self-appointed leaders wallowing in greed and deceit.'

As the TV blared into life, the screen revealed a smooth greasy egg, wearing gold rimmed spectacles. 'Oh no!' Sara screeched. 'It's the President of Vice!'

'Vice?'

'Vulgar Internationally Corrupt Evangelists.'

He was standing at the reception desk of a large plush office, surrounded by his entourage of Shushushu in dark glasses. Herded into the far corner by security guards was a motley crowd of very old people, thin, ragged, and dusty. The President of Vice was addressing a threadbare young man at the desk...

'Young man, why are you not looking after your aged parents? They have come here for their well-earned pensions, but you have given them nothing. I hereby order you to follow the Biblical commandment to honour your father and your mother, to respect your elders, and to pay these old people their pensions...'

At this point a wizened old woman broke free from her captors and threw herself at the feet of the President of Vice, washing his soft silver Italian shoes with her tears, and crying 'Oh Honourable Heavenly Saviour sent to us by God...'

Whereupon the President of Vice raised his hands to Heaven, crying out 'Help us Gaarhd!'

'Gaarhd?' I asked Sara. 'Is that the American pronunciation of God?'

'No,' said Sara, as the security guard came and threw the old woman back onto the pile. 'He was calling the Guard!'

The President of Vice seemed momentarily shaken by this attack upon his precious and perfumed person, pausing to mop his brow with a golden satin handkerchief.

'He must be very hot in that blue serge suit,' I said to Sara.

'Not at all, he's completely cold-blooded,' she laughed. 'That's hypocrisy oozing out through his skin.'

As if prompted by Sara's words, the President of Vice reached inside his jacket and took out a crocodile skin wallet. The starving pensioners fell to their knees in supplication, their hands raised eagerly towards the wallet. 'Let me see,' he said, 'whether I can alleviate the suffering of my people with a small donation.' But as he looked into the wallet a fatuous frown furrowed his fat face. 'Oh dear,' he said, 'I don't seem to have any local currency. I don't suppose you can accept American Express?'

As hope faded from the wallet, so all those assembled raised their hands towards Heaven, and the Voice of Vice slowly intoned 'We beseech you Oh Lord to restore the hard-earned pensions to these your miserable and humble servants!' Then, turning to the wretches themselves, and putting his handkerchief to his nose, he gave the sign of the cross and declared 'Your troubles are over, for the Lord will provide!'

So saying, he turned quickly on his heel, and stepped into his monstrous black Mercedes, and his convoy of twenty limousines went screaming away down the road in a cloud of dust, sirens blaring, as frightened citizens scattered respectfully into the ditch.

'Good gracious,' I said. 'How did this parasitic pastor become a member of the government?'

'He was appointed by God,' laughed Sara, 'Who, in his mighty and infinite wisdom, knows so much better than either the voters or the Constitution.'

'And why is the Pensions Board not paying the pensioners?'

'Because the government has looted all their money,' Sara laughed. 'How else do you think they managed to pay for those twenty limousines!'

'And does the President of Vice know all this?'

'Of course he does!' laughed Sara. 'He's not as stupid as he pretends!'

With the departure of the Voice of Vice, the TV news degenerated into its usual pattern of one deputy minister after another, each slowly and painfully trying to pronounce the long incomprehensible words written by their mischievous permanent secretaries.

But our attention was reclaimed by the announcer saying 'Here is a late news item which has just come in. The official residence of the President of Vice has been overrun by an army of pensioners, who say they intend to turn the vast mansion into an old people's home, and sell his twenty limousines in order to fund their missing pensions.'

'The Lord will provide,' laughed Sara.

'And from the International Airport,' continued the announcer, 'it is reported that the President of Vice is returning to Texas.'

'By American Express,' said Sara.

25th September 2003

4.5 Saved!

IT was past midnight at the Mega Music Disco, and I was lolling on the side bench, nursing a Whisky Black, as the rhumba vibration came up through the floor, reaching the parts that other music cannot reach. Suddenly towards me came a beautiful apparition squeezed into black tights, long braids swirling round her backless top. With one final silky swivel she landed herself neatly next to me, close and cosy.

'Nice to meet you,' I said, putting my arm around her, not wishing to appear unfriendly. 'My name's Kalaki, what's yours?'

'My friends call me Zambia,' she purred, 'because I get very hot in October.' She caressed my chin with her long silver fingernails. 'And I'm always attracted to men with beards.'

'Then we've nothing in common,' I said. 'I can't stand women with beards.'

She rubbed her chin against my cheek. 'Feel that,' she said. 'Smooth as a baby's bottom!'

'And is your bottom also as smooth as a baby's bottom?'

She put her lips to my ear, gave it a little nibble, and whispered 'That's for me to know and you to find out.'

But as we'd been talking, the music had stopped. 'What's going on?' I asked. 'The DJ has disappeared. Is it closing time?'

'It's time for the cabaret! That's what everybody's come for! Satire! Mumbo Jumbo the political clown, every night at this time, making the government look ridiculous!'

Just then the front door of the club burst open and there stood a podgy little Al Capone in black trilby hat and dark shades, his black leather coat billowing open to reveal a black satin suit, black shirt and black tie. He stood there poised in the doorway for a moment. Then he strode up to the bar, put his foot on the bar rail, and took off his hat with one dramatic sweep of his hand, revealing his face to the assembled company. 'It is I, the President of Vice!'

'Hurray!' laughed the crowd. 'Mumbo Jumbo is pretending to be the President of Vice! Come to save us from sin! So he can keep it all for himself!'

Mumbo Jumbo leant over menacingly towards the barman. 'Where is the owner of this establishment?' he roared.

The barman pretended to cower, whimpering 'He's gone to Tokyo, looking for investors.'

'Hah!' roared the Vice, 'nobody can believe a story like that! Obviously he's gone there to avoid me! I'm told you're operating without any licence whatsoever. I want to see your trading licence, tobacco licence, beer licence and liquor licence. Also your tavern licence, club licence, entertainment licence, import licence, and export licence. Also your work permit, pension fund registration, hygiene certificate, fire safety

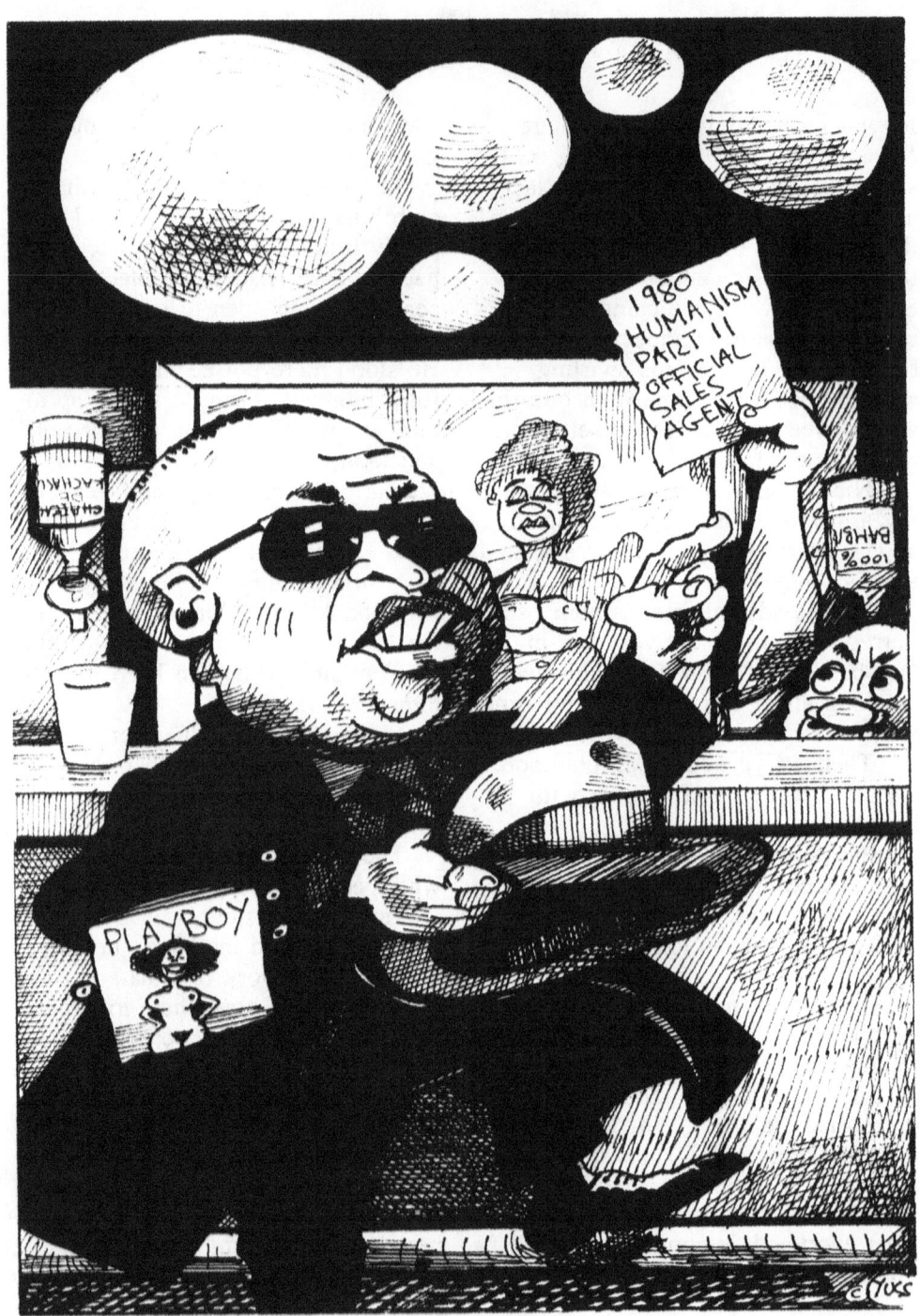

certificate and catering certificate. All of these things are important in order to encourage investors.'

The barman cringed, and slowly took a yellowed certificate off the wall. 'This is all we've got!'

'What! This is dated 1980, and licences you to sell Humanism Part II!'

'Yes, sir. We still have plenty left, if you'd like a copy.'

'For each of the fourteen missing licences you are fined 5 million, to be put in this hat!'

Then a voice from the crowd shouted out 'Hey, Vice, are you licensed to check licences?'

The Vice marched decisively to the microphone, taking a magazine out of his pocket and waving it high. 'Some people are questioning whether I myself am properly licensed. I shall therefore refer you to the Constitution.'

'That's a copy of Playboy,' somebody laughed, as the Vice opened the magazine.

'Some naughty boys may have played with it,' he said. 'But its all we have. It says here that any man who once fails in an erection shall never stand again.'

'And you failed!' we all shouted.

'For a time, yes,' explained the Vice, 'I did flop terribly, and felt I would never stand again. I felt terribly defeated, and rejected by everybody.'

'Yes,' Zambia whispered in my ear. 'Nobody wants a man who has flopped.'

'But after a time I rose up again, for the Lord says here on page 67 that a good man cannot be cast down for ever, but must always rise up. And so I threw off my feelings of defeat, and the Lord restored my self-confidence. And so it was that the Lord nominated me to come here today...'

'Ho ho,' laughed the crowd. 'Better than Tony Blair! Beware of his weapon of mass deception!'

'So now, by divine intervention,' continued the Vice, 'we don't need erections any more, with all their disease and corruption. For now I have been appointed by God to bring pure love to Zambia.'

'Oh Kalaki,' she said, holding me tight, 'Save me from all this!'

'Don't worry,' I said, as we scooted towards the door, 'Zambia shall be saved!'

2nd October 2003

Chapter 5
Wabufi Kafupi

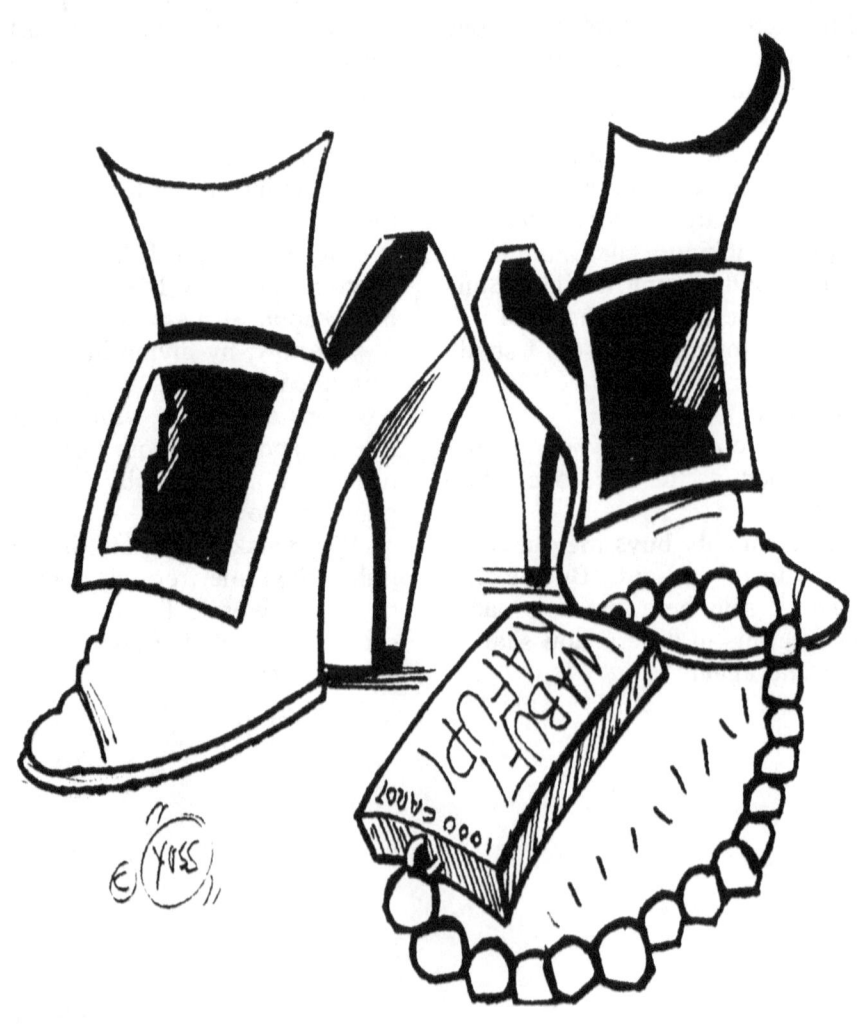

5.1 Forgive me, Father...

LAST week I found myself passing St Ignominious, and was tempted to go in, and have a look around. Automatically, I walked through to the back, into the little room where Sara and I once signed the marriage register, many years ago. I opened the door, and went in.

But now it seemed to be the confessional. A little wooden pew stood next to a metal grill in the wall. Curious, I opened the little side door, and stepped into the priest's secret little cubicle.

Very nice too! Comfortable red velvet armchair, bottle of whisky, and a Playboy magazine. I sat down, and poured myself a large glass of Jameson's Irish Whisky, and opened the magazine.

Just then I heard footsteps approaching on the other side of the grill. Then the steps came to a halt, and I could hear the visitor sitting down in the pew. My whisky hand began to shake. Next I heard a voice on the other side. 'Forgive me, Father, for I have sinned.'

I took another gulp at the whisky. 'Tell me, my son, what have you done which troubles your conscience?'

'Oh Father,' said the voice, 'I have chased my wife of many years, and now my house is empty.'

'A house without a wife is always empty,' I advised. 'You must turn your thoughts to God.'

'No, I mean the house is empty because she took all the furniture. She loaded everything into three containers, and took it all to Ndola. Not even a chair is left. That's why I have come here to sit down.'

'But my son, what did your wife do that you had to chase her, thereby accidentally chasing your furniture?'

'Father, she had become very moody and bad tempered, always trying to pick a quarrel with my other wives, and even criticising my choice of girlfriends.'

'Is that all, my son? You must explain to her that according to the Old Testament, a man may have many wives.'

'Its not as simple as that, Father. She has been seen with another man!'

'My son, that is an entirely different matter! Your wife has sinned. You must explain to her that the Bible allows a man to have many wives, but does not allow a woman to have many husbands. She has been unfaithful. That is adultery. A deadly sin.'

'So I did right to chase her?'

I lolled back in the armchair and took another gulp of whisky. 'My son,' I said, 'this is a Christian nation. You have to uphold the Old Testament rule that the man is the head of household. What troubles your conscience, apart from your dreadful loss of furniture?'

'Oh Father,' he wept, 'everybody is laughing at me. For I am the one who has talked about gender equality, but now people are saying I have one standard for myself, and another for my wife.'

I sat there admiring the centrefold of Playboy. 'My son,' I replied, 'women are biologically different from men. It is our duty to stay on top. Even in the Vatican, the Pope is always on top of the Mother Superior.'

'But Father,' he persisted, 'I have always tried to be a democrat. I have even written a book about democracy, which I intend to read one day. But now people are saying that I am a tyrant in my own home. Saying that I take decisions without consulting others. That I talk democratic and behave autocratic.'

'My son,' I said. 'You don't seem to know the true meaning of sin. Your only mistake is saying one thing, but doing another. You must drop all this hypocritical talk of gender equality and democracy, and make clear that you are following the Old Testament, the Dictatorship of God and the Tyranny of Man.'

'Thank you Father. What can I do to make amends?'

'Was that your first marriage?'

'No, second. Although I always called her my first lady.'

'Then you need to find a second lady, and go for a third term. On the way out, drop in at the Erectory and ask for Sister Magdelene. She's very experienced at uplifting the downcast. She could give you a marvellous erection for your third term.'

'What shall I tell her?'

'Tell her,' I said, 'to show you the true meaning of sin.'

I was still sitting there in a drunken stupor when the door of the cubicle opened, and there stood Father Fatty O'Flatulence. I drew myself unsteadily to my feet, and gave him the sign of the cross. 'Forgive me Father, for I have sinned.'

12th October 2000

5.2 Letter from the Bahamas

Dear Morleen,

Thanks for the lovely e-mail, giving all the news about your dear Kabeji. You know, my dear, when people used to talk about e-mail, I used to think they were talking about he-male. Of course you remember that I was just one of the cleaners, until my bottom got noticed. That was how I got poor Vera into so much trouble, by repeating her remark that she'd been connected to her hot-male for the whole night. That was when Kafupi turned to me for consolation. Ooh, my delicious littul Kafupi!

Anyway, my dear Morleen, here in the Bahamas I am still connected to my hot-male, and we're having a wonderful honeymoon. But I wonder how long it can last. You know the girls round here are walking around nekid. My little Kafupi's eyes have already started to wander. When the eyes start to pop out, the other parts will soon follow.

We are staying in the penthouse at the Carlington Hotel, which is owned by my littul Kafupi. He owns all the hotels on the island! And each of them is named after one of his naughty scandals. There's the Roan Palace, managed by the famous Binani Brothers, the Presidential Initiative managed by Slippery Sakala, and the five star Cobaltgate managed by Shameless Shamutete.

Did you know that all the time things were getting worse in Zambia, they've been getting better here in the Bahamas? Strange world, isn't it? The Bahamians have been getting fatter and living longer, with full employment, and free education and health care. No shortage of dollars here!

So sorry to hear all your rather depressing news from Zambia. Kafupi says don't worry about not having a majority in parliament. Just appoint Booby Bwalwa as Speaker. He can always be relied upon to announce that the ruling party has the majority of the votes cast.

And Kafupi says don't worry about the opposition refusing to vote for Bwalwa's appointment. All you have to do is to prevent five opposition members from voting. Kafupi says the best way is to instruct the Shushushu to leak information to these five, telling them that they are about to be arrested. Of course they will immediately blab to *The Post*. Then they can be arrested and charged with giving away state secrets, which is of course treasonable.

Don't try to explain all this to Kabeji. Just make your own phone calls to the Shushushu, DPP and IG telling them what Kabeji wants. Then write a little speech for him, in which he sternly emphasizes the enormity of their crimes, the unconstitutional means used, which threaten the security of the state, their contempt for democratic process, and the need for the full force of the law. He

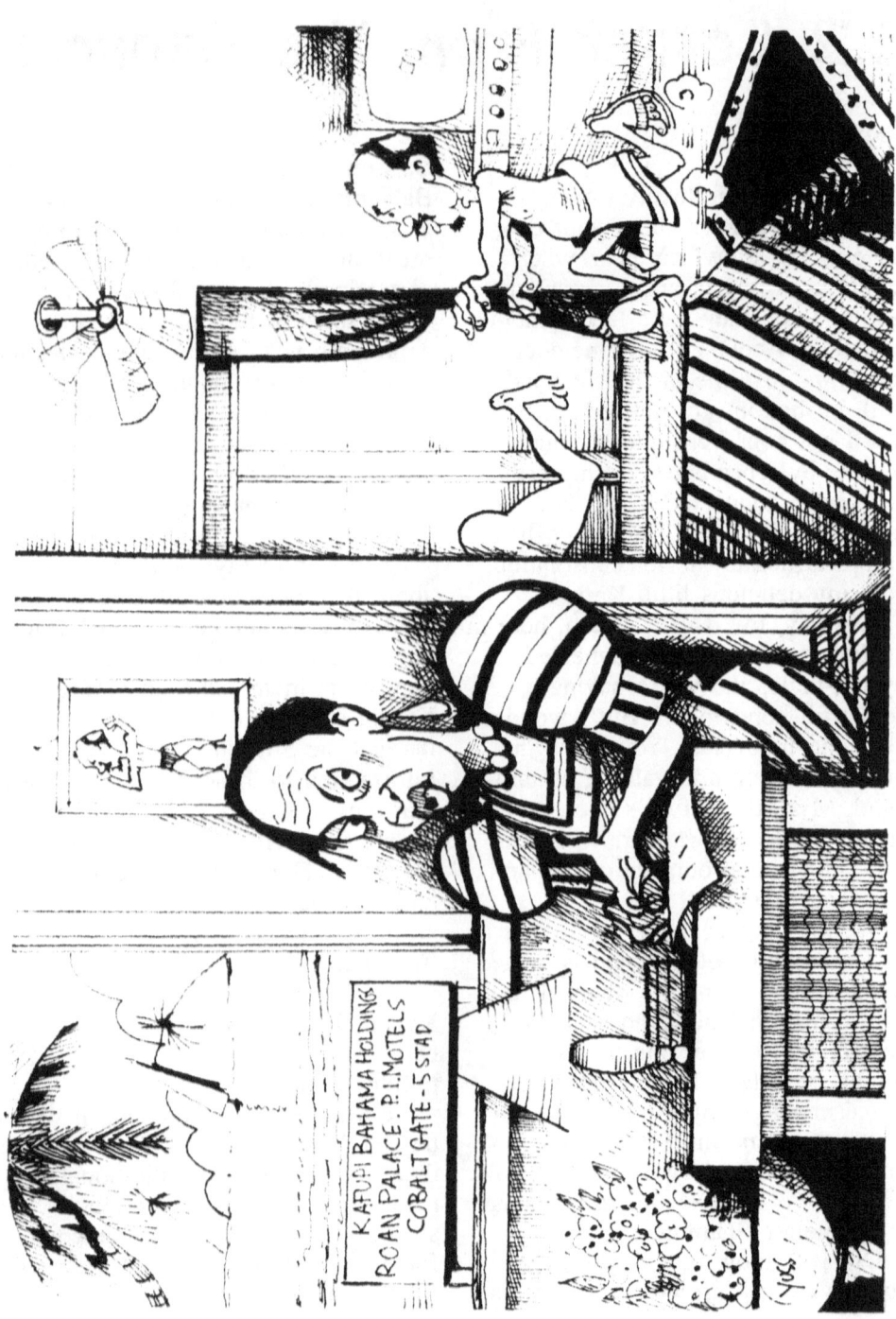

should explain that it's an offence for which the law does not allow bail, and it would not be right for him to interfere, the law must take its course. Blah blah, hah hah. You know the sort of thing. Kafupi left a list of essential phrases in the left hand draw of his desk. Just join these up to make a little speech. But he must practice saying 'constitutional'. He keeps saying 'constoowanal'.

Sorry to hear about the unpaid rates on Plot One, and the threats from Lusaka City Council to cancel the lease and take back the property. Kafupi says that under no circumstances can they be allowed to turn the place into a vegetable market. He says that the first person who brings a cabbage into Plot One must be arrested for disgracing the nation. A clear case of treason.

Kafupi also advises against reopening Yunza. We were very clear during the election that those who voted for the opposition would get nothing from us. We must keep our election promises. Anyway, this year's allocation for Yunza has already been put into the Bahama Dollar Account at the Zambia National Commercial Bank.

Kafupi is also annoyed about Kabeji promising to pay pensions. This is another sign that he hasn't understood his instructions. He has asked me to explain to you that party policy is to reduce life expectancy to thirty-five, after which nobody will be able to qualify for a pension. Therefore you should continue paying all pension contributions into the Bahama Account.

And lastly, one littul favour I ask of you, as a woman, my dear Morleen. Even as I write, my naughty littul Kafupi is giggling in the bedroom with a nekid chambermaid. I must get these girls at the Carlington Palace properly dressed, at least to cover their bottoms. Please send some party cadres down to Cairo Road to grab some girl's' trousers and skirts, and airfreight them here as soon as possible.

And Oh, I almost forgot! We wish both of you all the best in your fight against corruption.

Love, Regina.

17th January 2002

5.3 Paramount Thief

IT was the morning of Thursday 7 March 2003, and Sam and I were walking down the tree lined drive to the famous FTJ Institute at Kamfinsa, to attend the press conference of the famous Paramount Thief.

'Why FTJ?' I asked Sam. 'What's that stand for?'

'Back in the days of the Third Republic,' said Sam, 'this used to be Kamfinsa Prison, where all the worst criminals were sent. It became known as FTJ, the Famous Thieves Jail.'

'Amazing,' I said. 'And now its the centre of government.'

We walked through the entrance into the Great Hall, which was already full and buzzing with excitement. On one side were members of the diplomatic corps, and on the other side could be seen leading members of the Criminal Committee. Up front was Velvet Mango, Controller of Drug Trafficking, Godless Mandandu of Criminal Conspiracies, and Tricky Kawalala of the Prison Housing Initiative.

Then in swept the Paramount Thief, Wabufi Kafupi, surrounded by a small army of heavies. A tiny man, in purple zoot suit, with matching shades and high heel crocodile boots, he climbed up onto his high chair and reached up for the microphone. The cameras began to roll, as Zambia National Broadcasting for Criminals brought the pronouncements of the Paramount Thief to a fearful nation.

'Members of the diplomatic corps, fellow criminals and exploiters, I have invited you to my Institute today to explain the principles which underlie the process of democratisation in Africa.

'Those of you who have followed my career will know that the last time I called a press conference was more than a year ago, when I was still the Chief National Engineer and Architect. But shortly after that the Manda Hill Bridge collapsed, and my reputation and career collapsed with it. Despite my well known brilliance as an engineer, I had not designed the bridge to carry the enormous weight of the unexpectedly large number of tin trunks crossing the Great East Road from Parliament.

'But determined to start life again, I voluntarily gave away all my possessions, including houses and Mercs, and all the twenty-four cell phones which matched the different colours of my twenty-four suits. I was left with only the old bicycle on which I had originally arrived in Lusaka, back in 1991. So I cycled back to Ndola, to reconcile with my former wife.'

'He must have had a sore bum, after such a long ride,' Sam whispered.

'Perhaps she massaged his tender parts,' I suggested.

'Yes,' said Sam. 'That was when she realised that he still loved her.'

'I had to resume my career as a

tomato seller,' continued the Paramount Thief.

'But even this also ended abruptly when it was discovered that the tomatoes were stolen. So I voluntarily decided to come here to Kamfinsa, for a period of recuperation and philosophical reflection.'

'After receiving advice from a magistrate,' muttered Sam.

'It was here that I developed my ideas on kleptocracy, as an African version of democracy. According to the Western version of democracy, there should be a separation of power between the workers who produce the wealth, the executive who legally take their share, and criminals who illegally take theirs. In the West this works very well, because workers are many and productive, allowing massive capital accumulation by both government and criminals.

'But the West has tried to impose their system on us when we do not have enough wealth to go round. It causes workers to starve and the executive to become criminal, contradicting the separation of powers, and preventing capital accumulation. As we become poorer, so democracy becomes even more impossible.

'It was here in Kamfinsa that I realised that we cannot afford the wasteful parasites of the executive. We needed to develop a simple two-party system of workers and criminals, eliminating the executive.

'At Kamfinsa, this meant eliminating the prison warders. So first I invented a democratic system of the prisoners electing a Paramount Thief. We all agreed that prisoners with short sentences would cast only one vote, but those with long sentences would cast three. After that, I was easily elected as Paramount Thief, being particularly popular with the hard core criminals.

'Following the democratic principles of the free market, we privatised the prison under a management buyout, and sold all the prison bars to the Binani Brothers. Then we set up the place as the Kamfinsa Institute, to train criminals in how to run the country according to principles of democracy and good governance. The rest is history!'

We all stood up and cheered, as the heavies watched carefully for any sign of lack of enthusiasm.

'Hurray for the Paramount Thief!' they all shouted.

'Three cheers for the President!' I murmured.

'Don't call him that,' hissed Sam. 'You could be arrested!'

7th March 2002

5.4 The Settlement

'WHAT have we got this morning?' asked the Judge, as he sat himself on the bench.

'Divorce settlement for Mrs Dearer Kafupi, My Lord,' said the Clerk of the Court, as a woman in a brilliant green satin suit squeezed her ample bulk into the witness box. The morning sun glinted upon her many rows of pearls, and heavy duty gold earrings.

'My dear Dearer,' said the Judge, leaning forward and peering over his spectacles, 'What are you asking of this court?'

'My Lord,' said Dearer, 'my husband has divorced me, and left me destitute and starving.'

'I shan't ask you to swear on the Bible,' laughed the Judge. 'How much are you asking for?'

'For my share of the ploperty, My Lord.'

'Tell me about the marriage,' said the Judge. 'Did you help your husband in his work?'

'Oh yes, My Lord. When I met my littul Kafupi, he was just conductor on a littul minibus. That was more than thirty years ago. He had no qualifications at all. He only got the job because he was so short. He could walk up and down the minibus without having to bend.'

'So how did you help him make his money?' asked the Judge.

'I was the one who knew alithmetic. So I showed him how to count the money. And how to siphon off a little margin for himself.'

'So things began to go well?' suggested the Judge.

'Oh yes,' said Dearer. 'Soon we recluited all the other conductors into the same scheme, and set up the Movement for Marginal Diversion.'

'So all the conductors were on the take?'

'They all got their little share.'

'But your husband got more?'

'They all paid ten percent into his holding company, the Milking Money Deposit. He had the cheque book, but I was the blains behind it.'

'So how much would you say your husband is worth?'

'He's velly litch!'

'Just from milking the bus company?'

'That was only the beginning, My Lord. After milking the bus company, we soon moved into other organisations. We set up the Movement for Manipulating Democracy, for the diversion of government funds.'

'So you infiltrated the government?'

'More than that,' My Lord. 'We even managed to manipulate the Constitution.'

'But were you still assisting your husband, or was it him now doing all these things?'

'Oh no, My Lord. Without me it couldn't have worked. Sometimes it happened that a disgluntled gloup of people would become desperate and dangerous after Kafupi had diverted their wages, or pensions, or medicines. But then I would always alive by helicopter with a few bags of mealie meal for their empty bellies, some salaula for their naked bodies, and some salt for their wounds. Then they would jump and cheer, saying *Dearer was sent by Kafupi, and Kafupi was sent by God! Kafupi Mpusushi!'*

'What a marvellous marriage partnership!' declared the Judge. 'And a most equitable gender division of labour! For the Lord giveth, and the Lord taketh away! So what went wrong?'

'Sex,' said Dearer.

'Sex!' the Judge salivated. 'I've been waiting for this bit! Was he perverted? Insatiable? Bisexual? Was there any sadism? Masochism? Fetishism? Any whips? Black leather? Anything like that?'

'Don't over excite yourself,' snapped Dearer. 'It was just the normal sort of mid-life crisis. First his eyes began to wander. Then his hands began to wander. Then his other parts began to wander. He began to go with other women.'

'How many? Two at a time? Three at a time?' demanded the Judge, leaning forward, rubbing his hands, and bouncing up and down on his seat. 'Where did they do it? Did you catch them at it? Were they naked? Did you take any photos? Have you got any exhibits to put before the court?'

'Calm down, My Lord! For him, it was just a natural extension.'

'Natural extension? How big was his natural extension?'

'A natural extension of MMD, extended into Multiple Matrimonial Diversions. He used the helicopter to snatch other men's wives. Then he kicked me out of the house.'

'A thief and a philanderer!' gasped the Judge. 'How much is he worth?'

'About five billion dollars, My Lord.'

'Good God! And how much did you manage to carry away when you were chased?'

'Only a couple of million, My Lord. I'm destitute.'

'Well, Dearer, from what you have told me, I can see that you did your best to stick by your husband. Under the Matrimonial Causes Act of 1981, you are entitled to half of the marriage property. I therefore award you two and a half billion dollars.

'In addition, I sentence you to twenty years hard labour for receiving stolen property.'

18th April 2002

5.5 The Chosen One

SARA and I were sitting at the back of St Ignominious, as the fat bishop waddled to the podium to read the lesson to his thin and starving congregation. We were all gathered for the Thanksgiving for National Cleansing.

'The lesson this morning,' began the Bishop, 'is taken from the Book of Unbelievable Revelations, Chapter 23, Verses 1-12:

'And far beyond Judea there lay the land of Bupupu, which knew not the Lord, for it was a land of thieves. The streets were full of pickpockets and the markets full of stolen goods. A land where social status could not be achieved by wisdom nor good works, but only by the accumulation of stolen property.

'And the Lord was sorely troubled that his Commandments were being ignored, for in those days he liked to control everything. So he sent down the Archangel Gabriel, who appeared in a vision to a humble tomato seller, the talkative little Bwipi Kafupi.

'And the Archangel Gabriel spoke unto little Kafupi, saying *Verily I say unto you, the Lord has chosen you to lead your people out of the valley of sin and iniquity, into the chosen land of honesty and prosperity. You will become king and end all thievery in the land.*

And little Kafupi was much afraid, and answered unto the Archangel, saying *I am only a humble seller of stolen tomatoes, with small brain and long fingers. I am not worthy of this great task.*

'But the Archangel Gabriel spoke sternly unto him, saying *Know ye not that I am the one who impregnated your mother Mary while your father Joseph was busy with his girlfriend? You are therefore the Son of God, and must obey the commandments of your Father.*'

'What an unbelievable story,' I whispered.

'But not uncommon,' Sara chuckled. 'You should visit Chilenje Local Court!'

'And so it came to pass that Bwipi Kafupi was born again as the King of All Mpupu, for in those days the Lord's commands were taken very seriously. And so Kafupi sat on the big throne with his little legs dangling in the air, and the crown falling down over his little ears. But none of the citizens dared laugh, because they had great respect for the Lord and his Chosen One.

'And even little Kafupi soon became very devout, ending every sentence with *Allelujah* or *Praise the Lord*, for he was genuinely grateful that the Lord in his great wisdom had appointed such an unlikely candidate as King.

'But the King was sorely perplexed on how to use his small brain and long fingers to follow the Lord's commandment of ending thievery in the notorious land of Mpupu, where old traditions were much respected.

'But then one day, after much smoking of his favourite pipe, the king had a moment of divine inspiration. He saw that the answer to the problem was to take everything for himself. For if all wealth was held by the King, there would be nothing left for the people to steal, and their nasty habit of stealing would finally be ended.

'And so the King soon became known as Pompwe Kafupi, because he lived in such pomp and splendour, because everything belonged to him, while the people lived in misery and starvation. And the King always thanked God for his great fortune, saying *Bless me, O Lord, for these gifts which I receive by your Great Goodness, Amen*. And the people sang songs of praise for their King, for the King was very generous in rewarding all those who praised him.

'But the high priests and Pharisees became angry with the King, saying *Who is this King who has more money than the Church? To be given more praise than the Lord? And to have more girlfriends than the Bishop!'*

Their moral outrage rang out from the pulpits, until they incited a mob to storm the palace and drag the king before Pontius Pilate, shouting *Crucify him! Crucify him! He has stolen everything!*

'And Pilate replied calmly, saying *I can give you Jesus the carpenter or Kafupi the thief. Which do you choose?* But the mob was out of control, chanting *Crucify them both! They're in it together!*'

Now the Bishop looked up from the sacred text to explain further. 'So that is how Kafupi died. He took all the sin of theft upon his shoulders, that we might be cleansed. He died for us. Let us now stand up and sing Hymn 666, to the tune of *What a friend we have in Jesus* ...'

What a thief was Ba Kafupi
All our sins and grief to bear!
For he stole away our money
Everything for God in prayer!
O what peace he had to forfeit
O what needless pain to bear!
All that heavy guilt to carry
Everything for God in prayer!

18th July 2002

5.6 Sheriff's Sale
Advertisement in The Daily Sellout 3rd Oct 2002

Bankruptcy and Liquidation of Kafupi and Associates
Sheriff's Sale of Stolen Property

GOODS SPECIFIED IN THIS SCHEDULE HAVE BEEN SEIZED BY TASK FARCE BAILIFFS UNDER PROCESS IN ACTION NUMBER 01/2002/NEWDEAL/LEVY, BEING STOLEN PROPERTY NOW TO BE SOLD FOR CASH, AND THE PROCEEDS RETURNED TO THE RIGHTFUL OWNERS, THE PEOPLE OF ZAMBIA.

THE SPECIFIED GOODS WERE SEIZED FROM MUPUPU KAFUPI AND ASSOCIATES, NOW DECLARED BANKRUPT AND IN LIQUIDATION.

ALL GOODS LISTED IN THE SCHEDULE WILL BE SOLD BY PUBLIC AUCTION:

VENUE State House, Independence Avenue
DAY Thursday 3 October 2002
TIME 10.00 hours

GOODS LISTED IN THE SCHEDULE:

Furniture

One white leather armchair, too large for six small presidents, but too small for one large president. One purple plastic sofa, suitable for heavy duty encounters, needs new springs. One king size mattress/trampoline, ideal for multi-party sexual athletics.

Clothes and Personal Effects

275 Paris suits, high quality but very small, suitable for pompous pot-bellied dwarf. 4,321 pairs of high heel shoes, all expensive but extremely vulgar, suitable for Emelda Marcos, and other tacky gear too numerous to mention.

Books and Documents

Twenty copies of *The Rule of Law* by Prof. Muna Ndulo, untouched and still in the original plastic wrapping. One copy of a master's thesis on democracy, author unknown. One million presidential ballot papers (already marked). Two copies of the *Gabon Report*, both bloodstained.

Logistical Equipment

Two thousand ballot boxes (already stuffed). Two hundred tin trunks (empty). Ten kilometres of tunnel, with no light at the other end, suitable for use during a popular uprising.

Pick-up Trucks

120 Mazda pick-ups, mysteriously picked up from nowhere, with money

picked up from somewhere, and very useful for picking up votes from nowhere.

Other Transport Vehicles

One V-24 fuel injection Jaguar Supercar, one BMW high-speed motorbike, one Challenger speedboat, and one Apache helicopter, all left behind by the Mastermind of Top Intelligence when he tried to flee the country on a bicycle.

Real Estate

130 huge mansions, built by Malumba and Kachungwa, and situated in Lusaka, Chienge, Chilubi Island and the Bahamas. Particularly suitable for storing girlfriends, concubines, tin trunks, and fugitives from justice. Copies of title deeds can be obtained from Swindle Mulenga and Associates, Photocopiers.

Mine Shaft

One large empty hole in Luanshya, ideal for disposing of rioting copper miners, and any other malcontents and rabble rousers who threaten the property of respectable citizens.

Former Employees of Kafupi

One Chief Justice, quite expensive to bribe, more suitable for judicial systems in Colombia or Nicaragua. One Auditor General, can be bought very cheap. One wooden Vice-President, very durable, but well past his sell-by date. One Chief Clerk, never properly qualified, but very experienced in petty theft and poaching. One unspeakable Speaker, blind and deaf, and therefore completely immune to shame, but still with dangerous teeth. Plus many other worthless parasites too numerous to mention.

METHOD OF PAYMENT

All bids must be made in dirty brown envelopes, available from Cycle Mata. All payment must be in cash, delivered in tin trunks. All cash should be in dollars supplied by the Bank of Zambia. Dollars supplied by Francis Nkhoma are not legal tender.

SALE PROCEEDS GO TO STARVING ORPHANS

Proceeds from this sale will be used to pay the expenses of the Morleen Mwanamwana Initiative, to send a delegation to Paris to attend the Starving Orphans Charity Ball.

SIGNED:

Kalaki

Inspector Kalaki
Leader of the Task Farce

5.7 Vera's Story

I knocked on the front door of the little house in Twapia, and it flew open straight away. 'Karaki!' Exclaimed Vera, throwing her arms around me. 'I haven't seen you since the days of the Gleen Libbon! Come in! With your beard and long shirt and fat belly, I thought it was the Archbishop of Canterbury! What has been happening to you?'

'I was impregnated by Milingo,' I laughed, 'so I had to join the church! But never mind me, I've come to talk to you about your ex, and his present troubles. How did he ever get himself into such a pickle?'

'It's a long story,' she sighed. 'Come and sit down and I'll tell you everything.'

'What puzzles me,' I said, as we sat down together on the purple plastic sofa, 'is how we voted for him to bring democracy and end corruption, and he did the opposite. He seemed so straightforward, but now it seems he had his fingers in every till. Its almost like he turned into another person.'

'You know, Kalaki,' she said, putting her hand on mine, 'you seem to have a nose for things. I've always said you're not as silly as you look. Let me tell you what actually happened, when we first moved into the Presidential Palace. I can still remember that Thursday morning, as if it were yesterday. The place was so huge, and my little Fleddie was so small, and when lunch was ready we couldn't find him.'

'But you eventually found him?'

'Yes, three hours later, in one of the upstairs toilets, reading a book. Do you know that place has thirty-four toilets?'

'What was he reading?'

'Humanism,' laughed Vera. 'Old Munshumfwa had taken all the other books, only Humanism remained, in all the lavatories.'

'There was a terrible shortage of toilet paper in those days,' I reminded her. 'That's how the Second Republic ended, with Humanism being flushed down the toilet.'

'So is that what changed him, reading the toilet paper?'

'No,' she said, as tears welled into her eyes. 'It was much worse than that. Two days later he disappeared again, and this time we couldn't find him at all. We never found out what happened. Whether he had fallen into one of the tunnels, or had been blown up the chimney, or flushed down a toilet, or eaten by a peacock. My poor littul Fleddie was gone!'

'But this wasn't reported in the papers!'

'Of course not! Causing public alarm is a climinal offence. We had to keep it quiet!'

'And was he never found?'

'Two weeks later he turned up on the doorstep. Or at least it seemed to be him, except that he was wearing a salaula suit, sunglasses, barbie doll high heels, and speaking with a weird American accent. He had changed tellibly!'

'And I said *Darling you're back! Come and have a bounce on the purple plastic sofa!* But he seemed to have forgotten everything. He jumped on the sofa and started to trampoline all by himself, until he made this hole with his high heel,' she said, pointing to the punctured purple plastic right next to where I was sitting.

'My poor dear,' I said, putting my arm round her. 'Your best sofa!'

'And my Fleddie had always had this delicious littul mole on his lovely littul bum. But when we went to bed,' she sobbed, 'there was no spotty on his littul botty!'

I put my arm around her, as she wept into my cup of tea. 'How could this have happened?'

'You see, my littul Fleddie Mpundu was a twin. Now the other one, Kafupi, had turned up to take his brother's place. A rascal and ne'er-do-well. A former tomato seller and bus conductor! And now my husband!'

'How could he do that?'

'In my tradition, the brother inherits the widow.'

'But didn't people in government notice that this was not the right man?'

'Because of his high office, they just had to obey his instructions, however silly! Its all explained in the Constootion.'

'But can he be held responsible for all his mistakes?'

'I'm sure he had no idea what he was doing, he was always in a cloud of smoke. That's why he has even asked the Task Farce to find out whether he ever went to the Bahamas. He never had any idea where he was, what he was doing, or where the money went.'

'But can we prove that this man is not the real Fleddie?'

'I've told you!' she sobbed. 'No spotty on his botty! He must be undressed in public!'

'What have you been doing today?' asked Sara, when I finally got home.

'I've just heard a fantastic story from Vera,' I said, 'about how her husband completely changed into somebody else!'

'Huh!' said Sara. 'All women have that problem.'

27th February 2003

5.8 Death Trap

I scanned the sea of empty chairs in the vast sitting room. Nobody there at all. I was just about to leave when I spotted the wrinkled and diminutive Kafupi Kadoli, sitting up like a cocky cockroach in the corner of a huge white leather armchair. 'Kafupi!' I said, as I went over to greet him, 'Where is everybody? Have all your friends deserted you?'

'Certainly not!' he laughed, 'They're all down at the magistrate's court, where my case is coming up later this morning. Do excuse me for not standing up to greet you, but its such a struggle to climb back up onto this chair.'

'That's life,' I said. 'Once you slip down, its always difficult to climb back. Maybe you could apply to the Physiotherapy Department to be given a little ladder.'

'Certainly not!' he snapped. 'I've always been against government assistance for the handicapped. Anyway, Kalaki, what brings you here today? To talk about ladders?'

'Of course not,' I laughed. 'I came to ask you about the Aeroplane Disaster of 1993.'

'Hah! Nowadays *The Post* seems to be entirely preoccupied with resurrecting corpses from ten years ago. Maybe you should change the paper's name to *The Postmortem*.'

'Were you the one responsible for the crash?'

'Hah! Certainly not! I have a perfect alibi! I was on an official trip to Bujumbura at the time of the disaster. Four thousand kilometres from the scene of the crime!'

'But you were in Lusaka when the decision was taken to use the ill-fated aircraft. So you must be implicated.'

'Certainly not!' he retorted. 'That was two days before it happened, and two thousand kilometres away from where it happened. So how could I have been involved?'

'It is claimed that the aircraft was a Death Trap.'

'Certainly not! It was a Blundering Bugaboo, made in Canada in 1923.'

'But were you not the one who took the decision to use this ancient old Bugaboo?'

'Certainly not! The decision was taken by the officer in charge of all our Blundering Bugaboos, Air Marshall Shaky Shikashiwa.'

'Perhaps he advised against using the plane, and you overruled him?'

'Certainly not! I ruled over him, but I didn't overrule him.'

'But you demanded blind loyalty?'

'Certainly not. I allowed him to open his eyes and have a look at the plane.

'He reported that one wing was loose. Wasn't that dangerous?'

'Certainly not! I made a point of showing him the spare wing on the other side.'

'Is it true that one engine was getting too hot?'

'Certainly not! Engines are supposed to get hot.'

'Since you left earlier for Bujumbura, I wonder why you didn't use the Blundering Bugaboo? If it was such a nice plane, wasn't it also suitable for you?'

'Certainly not. My wife was far too large to fit through the small door of the Bugaboo. So reluctantly we had no choice but to use the luxury Boeing 737.'

'So the Bugaboo wasn't a Death Trap?'

'Certainly not.'

'So you don't feel responsible for the death of the Fallen Heroes.'

'Certainly not, Kalaki. In fact, that would be logically impossible. You see, it is only possible to become a Fallen Hero after death, so nobody can cause the death of a Fallen Hero. Perhaps you meant to ask whether I should feel responsible for turning these young men into Fallen Heroes.'

'And do you?'

'Certainly not! It was the outpouring of national grief that turned them into Fallen Heroes. I certainly wouldn't want to claim any special responsibility for that. Although I was careful to make sure that I wept more than anybody else.'

'It was a national tragedy.'

'Certainly not. It provided a marvellous national re-awakening. It brought us all together as a nation after a period of political division and acrimony.'

'But it was also a time of much murmuring that our leaders did not care for the people's heroes, and negligently sent them to their fate in a rickety old Death Trap. That must have been a great embarrassment to the government.'

'Certainly not! Simply not true! On the contrary, people understood that it was not the business of government to be providing air transport. They soon understood that government funds were meant only for government leaders, and not ordinary citizens, who should pay for themselves.'

'To stay alive?'

'Certainly not. Since the Fallen Heroes, people have now become more accustomed to mass funerals. Nowadays we assist people in passing quickly to Heaven, to re-unite with their Fallen Heroes.'

Just then Kadoli's secretary put his head round the door. 'The Minister for Shushushu, Air Marshal Shaky Shikashiwa, has sent a limousine for your trip to court. Its already waiting outside. Shall I tell the driver to wait?

'Certainly not!' screamed Kafupi. 'It might be a Death Trap!'

4th December 2003

Chapter 6
Vera's Diary

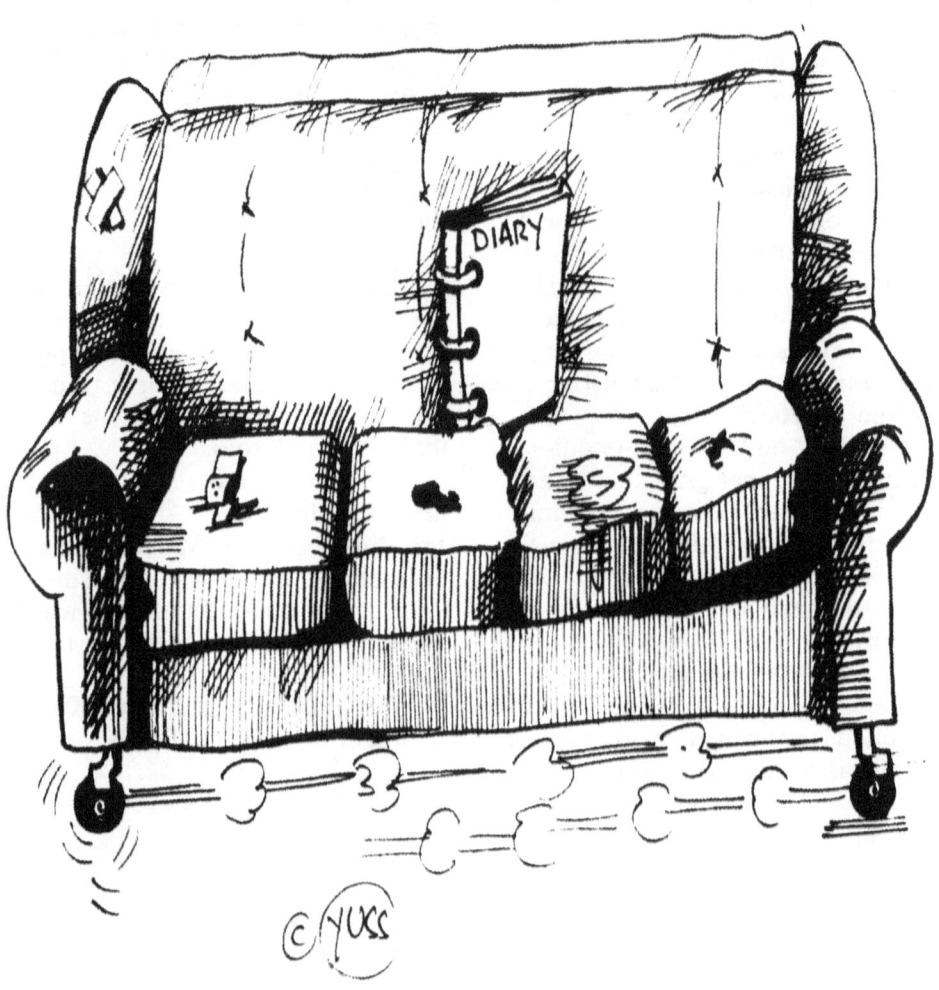

6.1 The Auction

Friday 3 May
Dear Diary, Today the auctioneer, Mr Selloff Figov, came to arrange for tomorrow's auction. I'm selling off everything, even my purple plastic sofa.

Not everybody knows, *Dear Diary,* the secrets of my Kadoli and our purple plastic sofa. It all began when I was a young girl in Twapia. I did so much want to have a husband of my own, but no man came for me.

So that was when I made my own littul man for myself, my littul Kadoli. And while the other girls were playing with their men, I was playing with my own littul Kadoli on my own purple plastic sofa. How we bounced up and down! Because of my belief in him, he finally became a real man, who could stand up for himself!

My littul Kadoli made me happy in so many ways. After I powered him with four Mansa batteries he was a very convincing littul fellow. Talked beautifully, with words I taped from the BBC. No real human feelings of course. Absolutely heartless. But you can't have everything!

He would go and collect anything for me, his dear darling. A tiny little fellow who could pass straight between any burglar bars. His dinky littul feet left no footprints. And his fingers, much longer than his littul legs, could reach into any till. What more could any wife want?

I even used to dress him up as a plesident, so he could visit his counterparts all over the world, and nick all the best bits from their palaces. They never suspected he was just a common thief!

But I made him too luvely. Other women began to fancy him. Now I am left here all alone, with no choice but to sell off my beautiful things. The auction is tomorrow.

Saturday 4 May
Dear Diary, it started off so well! A big clowd of people, and Figov was marvellous.

He sold off the DVD player, the one with all the knobs and buttons! I never did find out how to play it! He sold the 205 inch gold TV, the platinum satellite dish, and all my Persian rugs, for millions of gluders. All cash, pushed straight into his black leather bag.

The first sign of twouble came with the big clystal chandelier in the sitting room. You know, the one that hangs right down to the floor, and covers the coffee table.

'A genuine imitation grass chandelier from Carnival Furnishers!' shouted Figov. 'How much am I offered!'

Some fat bling bling from New Kasama had just offered a million gluders when some stiff shirted burwokwat held up a bit of paper and said 'Harf a minit, I have a court injunction lestraining the sale. I have information that this is a genuine

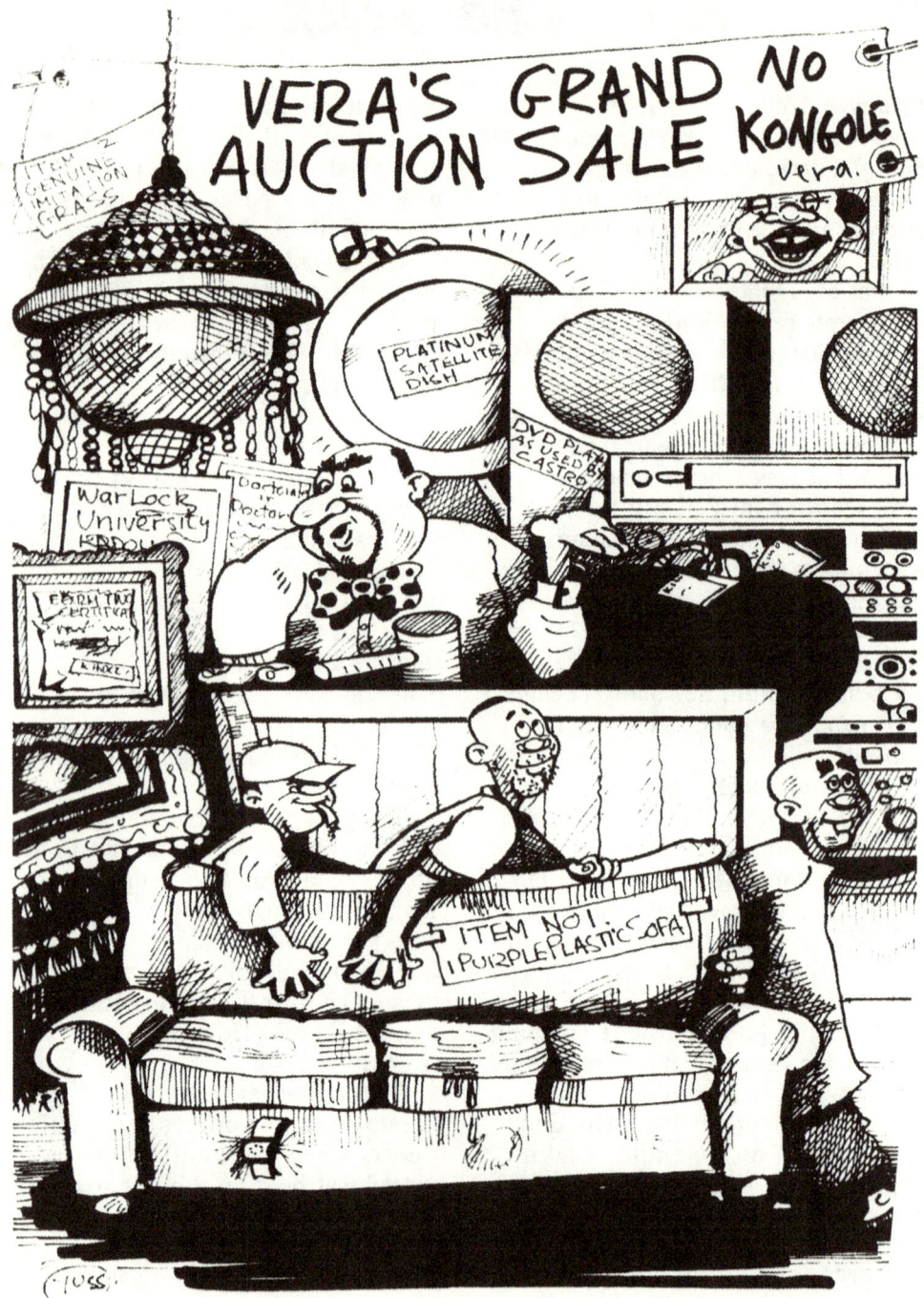

Louis XIV chandelier stolen from the Versailles Palace in 1998!'

But things went better when we came to my Kadoli's beautiful certificates. Figov introduced them nicely, saying 'These are the three certificates that made Kadoli believe that he was a real person, and made him what he is today. The first one is the famous forged Form Two certificate that is credited with increasing the sales of Tippex correcting fluid throughout the Commonwealth. The second is the Masters Degree in Wizardry from Warlock University, which unfortunately caused the fall of that ill-fated institution. Lastly we have this marvellous Doctorate in Doctoring, which certifies Kadoli's ability to doctor any document.'

Everybody shouted 'Three cheers for the Paramount Thief!' as the certificates were sold for a thousand gluders to Transparency International, who want them for their new Museum of Corruption in New York. I felt so ploud!

Then everybody went into the garden to look at the S500 Merc. But again things went wrong when a seedy little gnome stepped forward, saying 'I am Bigwig Abashi, and this vehicle belongs to the Ministry of Worms for Supply. As the Chief Worm, it has been allocated to me!' Then he got in it, and drove off!

Figov was marvellous, pretending nothing was wrong. He turned to the crowd and said 'Never mind that! The best is yet to come!' as four men carried my prize purple plastic sofa into the garden. But guess what! My littul Kadoli was sitting in the corner of the sofa!

I screamed and fainted. When I woke up, everybody was looking down at me, saying 'Poor Dear! You're alright now!'

But Kadoli had escaped in the confusion! Completely gone! And so had Figov's black bag! After all that, I was left with nothing!

'Never mind,' said my old friend, Spectator Kalaki, as he sat with me on the purple sofa and put his arm round me. 'You're an independent woman now. You can earn your own money. You can write for *The Post*!'

2nd May 2002

6.2 All is not lost!

Saturday

Dear Diary, its been five weeks since I moved into my littul house in Twapia. So quiet and peaceful. What a relief to be free of all those bootlickers trying to wangle favours out of littul Fleddie. I'll be too happy if I never see that Slippery Sata again.

Just like old times, sitting on the same littul, Furncoz chairs which we bought back in 1982. All those big puffy purple chairs I bought from Manda Hill, they're still sitting outside. I can't get them in through the littul door.

My Fleddie always insisted this was a big house, but I always said it was small. That's when we first began to quarrel.

Sunday

Who should drop in this morning, but my old friend Valentine Kadopy, to show me his new wife Bella. How embarrassing! It's the same problem with all this puffy stuff from Manda Hill! We couldn't get him in through the front door. So we had to sit outside, on the purple plastic.

Poor old Valentine fell asleep straight away, so I was able to have a nice chat with Bella. 'How do you like the cumbersome old monster?' I asked.

'What?' she said. 'The sofa?'

'No,' I laughed, 'Valentine. You'll never be able to control him. Couldn't you have found something smaller?'

'He's no trouble at all,' laughed Bella. 'During the day he's so busy with foreign affairs that he comes home exhausted. So he doesn't interfere with me at all. It's the first time in years that I've been able to get a good night's sleep.'

'He has the reputation of sleeping with everybody,' I said, as we looked at the Incredible Bulk, sunk deep in the purple sofa.

'Yes,' laughed Bella. 'If the *Monitor* gets hold of this story, they'll say he's sleeping with both of us!'

Monday

Dear Diary, look at *The Post* this morning! This Laurence Kalaliki, the man from World Bankrupt, has been shedding crocodile tears over the starving children in Maheba. Isn't he the very one who caused our poverty in the first place? Maybe he was crying because they weren't fat enough to eat.

Do not worry, dear children. Soon I shall revive my Dope Foundation and chase these reptiles back to the Washington Zoo.

Tuesday

I worry about poor Fleddie, trying to struggle on without me. Most people didn't realise that I was the one taking all the decisions. My littul Fleddie always came home in a terrible muddle from those Cabinet meetings. 'All that talk,' he would say, 'and everybody in favour of doing something different. Now I don't know what to do!'

'Take no notice of all of them!' I would say. 'You're the Big Man! So be a man! Be the Boss! Change the Constitution!'

At night he would cry himself to sleep on my bosom. But the next morning he would wake up confident and decisive. 'I've had a great idea,' he would say. 'I shall change the Constitution!'

So that's how it went. *'Arrest them! Release them! Appoint them! Expel them!'* I was the one who gave him all the big ideas.

Wednesday

Dear Diary, cheeky letter in *The Post* this morning from somebody called Chongo Chiluwelubwe, saying I have spare time to record gospel songs, and for Spectator Kalaki to publish my diaries.

How I wish I could retire! But I have to get back! Have you seen how the country is going to the dogs since I left? Petrol up! Kwacha down! Children starving! More crocodile tears from Mack Dimwit!

But do not worry, *Dear Diary,* I shall save us from the crocodiles! I am the only one who can save the nation. That's why Fleddie became suspicious when I told him not to go for a third term. He thought I was going for a third term without him. That's why he suspected me of being unfaithful, and put Slippery Serpent to spy on me.

It's because he's called Slippery Serpent that people think he's a snake. So when I had a friend called Archie Matrimony, everybody thought he was my husband! So the Serpent expelled me from the party. Then Fleddie expelled me from the house! *Naimwe, BaFleddie bawishi Castro*!

Which was just as well, because now I can go for a third term. I intend to go Up and Down with Randy Bazooka! I shall be the First Lady again! Just as soon as I can get this Lumpy Kadopy off my purple plastic sofa!

So no time for recording gospel songs! And I shall never allow Spectator Kalaki to publish my Diary!

Do not worry, Ba Chongo, all is not lost!

9th November 2000

6.3 Flee at last!

Sunday

Dear Diary, what a surprise this morning when my dear little Fleddie paid me a visit. Nobody had recognised him arriving on his bicycle, dressed as a tomato seller. I gave him such a tight hug that I squashed his tomatoes. Just like the old days!

Its terrible the way we have to meet in secret like this, since I returned to our littul house in Twapia to prepare for our retirement. I told Fleddie at the time, I said just tell them the truth, that you're not going for a third term. But he didn't know how to tell them. Instead he invented a story that we had separated after a bust-up.

Fleddie, I said, nobody will believe a story like that. We've been known as such a God-fearing Christian couple, always sitting on the front row in church, and lecturing others on being faithful. Anyway, who would believe that such a little fellow could chase a big woman like me!

But Fleddie just laughed, saying people always believe stories when they're more horrible. That's why the Crucifixion has always been so popular.

Oh my delicious little tomato, he's too clever!

Monday

For his breakfast I gave him his usual mealie meal porridge, on his favourite blue enamel plate that we bought all those years ago at the OK Bazaar. And the yellow plastic table cloth with the pink flowers, that always used to brighten him up in the good old days. But this morning he was very glum and glumpy.

I put my arm around him and gave him a squeeze, as a big tear rolled into his porridge. 'Just tell them you're leaving the job,' I said. 'Then you'll be flee. Flee from that awful job. Its too much for you. They'll understand.'

'They won't,' he sighed. 'I appointed them all!'

'They'll be able to find other jobs.'

'That's the problem,' he moaned. 'I appointed only fools who would do exactly what I demand without question. Mindless loyalty. Without me, they're completely un-employable.'

(But don't worry, *Dear Diary!* I have devised a plan to flee my littul Fleddie! Just wait and see what happens tomorrow!)

Tuesday

Fleddie was still scowling at his breakfast porridge when there was a knock at the door. 'Yes! What is it!' he shouted, as he flung open the door, and found a large kaponya with a *Chiluba Wamuyayayayaya* slogan all over his shirt.

'I'm Mike Shushu,' the kaponya shouted back. 'Of NOCE, the National Organisation for Constitution

Eradication. This is the SSS.'

'What's that mean?' laughed Fleddie. 'Shushushu?'

'No, a Selected Sample Survey,' said Shushu. 'First I need to know whether you are an MP, district administrator, or party official.'

'Party official,' replied Fleddie.

'Good' said Shushu. 'Then I have a couple of questions for you. Firstly, do you think that a president who has not completed his programme should be given another term in office?'

'Good gracious no!' laughed Fleddie. 'Failure to complete a programme should obviously be a good reason for choosing somebody else!'

'Just one more question,' said Shushu. 'Should we change the Constitution to allow a president to stay in office indefinitely?'

'Certainly not,' shouted Fleddie. 'I have always said we must set the limit at two terms, to avoid returning to dictatorship. I'd look very silly now, if I said anything different! Thank you and goodbye!'

Fleddie slammed the door in his face, and turned to me. 'Ah my little pumpkin, I feel better after getting that off my chest! Let's go and sit on the purple plastic sofa!'

Wednesday

Dear Diary, everything has gone according to plan. This morning I found a letter pushed under the front door. When my eyes fell on its beautiful words, I knew I had saved my littul Freddie ... *Suspended from the Party with immediate effect ... gross indiscipline ... write exculpatory letter ... to be received by yesterday at the latest ... return the bicycle immediately.*

'Fleddie!' I shouted, 'Good news! You're off the hook!'

We were still standing there rejoicing when the door flew open with a bang, to reveal twenty-five armed paramilitary. 'Is this the home of Titus Tomato Kafupi?' one of them shouted, holding up my Fleddie's littul bicycle. 'He's under arrest for being in possession of stolen property!'

'Don't you worry, my precious tomato!' I shouted after my littul Fleddie, as they threw him into the back of the lorry. 'Your troubles will soon be over! And give my love to Archie!'

But in the meantime, *Dear Diary,* I'm all alone again on my purple plastic sofa.

29th February 2001

6.4 The Gleen Libbon

Sunday

Poor lonely me. I have only you, *Dear Diary,* to talk to. Only you can know how lonely I am in my littul house here in Ndola. Forgive me, *Dear Diary,* if my tears fall on you.

Nowadays I cannot bear to sit on my purple plastic sofa. It brings back those memories of how we used to bounce together. Instead I sit on my littul stool and weep. Every morning I polish my purple plastic sofa with cobra, just as I used to rub him all over with soap. An act of love for a missing husband.

Never did I think, when we moved to that big house in Lusaka, that it would all come to this. What went wrong? Why did he chase me? I still don't understand.

Monday

So near but yet so far! Tonight I saw my littul Kafupi on the TV. Everybody loves my littul Kafupi. I moved the TV onto the purple plastic sofa, so I could sit next to my darling, and give him a big hug.

He was handing out brown paper envelopes to everybody. Then off they all went, marching and singing a song. It sounded like *Turd turn! Turd turn!* I couldn't understand it at all.

Tuesday

What a dreadful day! My world has been turned upside down! This morning when there was a knock on the door, I thought my littul Kafupi had come back to me. But it was his Uncle Ben. 'How is he?' I asked. 'Have you brought any message? I saw him on the TV last night!'

'That's the problem,' said Ben. 'That wasn't really Kafupi Mpundu. It was his twin brother Wabufi Mpundu!'

'What!' I exclaimed. 'I was told that his twin died at birth!'

'Kafupi always disowned his delinquent brother,' explained Uncle Ben. 'But they're both alive alright. One twin grew up to be your husband, the distinguished Dr Kafupi Mpundu, world authority on democracy and honesty in politics. The other grew up to be Mr Wabufi Mpundu, the notorious trickster, manipulator, liar and thief. Identical in appearance, but opposite in virtue. That's why, traditionally, newly born twins were left in the forest to die. Because nobody could tell which one was the work of the Devil.'

'Oh My God! This evil Wabufi has taken the place of my dear Kafupi! So that's why I was banished here to Ndola! Because I am the only one who knows the naughty place of my dear littul Kafupi's birthmark! But what has Wabufi done with him? Dumped him in the forest? Uncle Ben, why haven't you reported Wabufi to the police?'

'You know the old saying in Luapula,' he smirked. 'Blood is thicker than sewage.'

Wednesday

Another knock on the door this morning, and again I thought my dear littul Kafupi had come back to me. But it was a man selling gleen libbons. 'What for?' I asked.

'Its the Gleen Levolution,' he explained, 'we're trying to save our environment from pollution.'

'Are we in danger?'

'Oh yes,' he replied. 'Some nasty little turds in Lusaka are trying to pollute the environment. They want to bring back everything smelly and nasty, and parade it in the street. Even the sewage we thought we had flushed away, they want to bring it back for reprocessing. They are trying to stir the shit! They are called the Turd Turners!'

'So how does the gleen libbon help?'

'You wear your gleen libbon in the shape of a cross, to protect yourself from the Devil. If any Turd Turner tries to pollute you, just show him your gleen libbon. Instead of turning you into a Turd Turner, the Turd Turner will turn back into a turd.'

Thursday

Another knock on the door! I look out the window, but there's nobody to be seen. Then it must be my little Kafupi, come back at last! But first I rush to arrange the cushions on the purple plastic sofa, and undo the top button on my blouse. But then panic! Suppose its Wabufi! I don't want Kafupi to accuse me of being unfaithful! So I quickly glab the gleen libbon and pin it to my blouse. Then rush back to the door, and fling it open!

'Kafupi?' I said. 'Is it really you? My darling?'

But as he leant forward to give me a kiss, his eyes fell on the gleen libbon.

'Aaarrghh!'

He fell down in agony, then disappeared in a cloud of smoke. Nothing left except a small brown mess on the mat.

Amazing what a gleen libbon can do!

8th March 2001

6.5 The Exorcist

Tuesday

Dear Diary, it seems so long since I came here to Twapia to prepare our littul house for our retirement. I sit here looking at our beloved purple plastic sofa, so full of romantic memories. I look at the spring sticking out of the middle cushion, and remember our last wedding anniversary. What painful ectasy! What a man, my littul Fleddie!

But it was a tellible mistake to leave my poor dear littul Fleddie all alone in that big house in Lusaka, haunted by ghosts and evil spirits. Now he is trapped by devils and demons, all led by Old Beelzebub himself, the dreaded Michael Satan.

My husband is such a good man, but he is surrounded by evil. Oh my lovely Fleddie, how can I get you out of there?

Wednesday

This afternoon I had a visit from Fleddie's old fiend, Clismar Tembo. He has lun away from the haunted house, and is welly wullied about my Fleddie. He says Fleddie's big mistake was to declare a Christian Nation. This has encouraged all the devils in the world to congregate in Lusaka, to try to defeat God's work. He's so good and innocent, my Fleddie. He doesn't realise how much evil there is in the world.

Clismar has invited me to join his new committee, the Forum for Destroying Devils, the FDD. One of the White Fathers, St Simon Righteous, has agreed to serve as chairperson. We're going to save my Fleddie from the evil spirits!

Thursday

My *Dear Diary*, I'm so excited, St Simon has worked out a plan for saving my Fleddie. He's bringing back Archbishop Immaculate Milungu to exorcise all the devils! St Simon says Milungu is so good at it that the Pope once gave him the job of exorcising all the devils from the Vatican. It took him more than twenty years. Apparently there were more devils than cockroaches.

So now he's coming back to Zambia to save us, and to rescue my little Fleddie. He's going to be given my littul Fleddie's job as Chief of the Christian Nation, so he can drive all the devils out of government. Then my darling will be able to retire, and come back to me.

I have already phoned the man at Carnival Furnishers, to come and mend the spring in the purple plastic sofa. I don't want to damage my lovely littul Fleddie.

Friday

Oh *Dear Diary*, things are going wrong. *The Post* has got wind of the story to put the Archbishop in charge. That Meddlesome Mercutio claims that all the nuns in Zambia consider themselves as wives of the Archbishop. And then there is the problem of all the childless women who visit the Immaculate Milungu, so that he can give them immaculate conception.

The Post editorial has argued that these religious duties will leave the Archbishop completely exhausted, and he won't have any energy left to serve as Chief Executive of the Christian Nation.

One First Lady is enough says *The Post*. I quite agree.

Saturday

Dear Diary, my Fleddie would be so ploud of me. This afternoon the Executive Committee of FDD met in my littul sitting room. We were working out a way to save my littul darling, still trapped in Lusaka with nobody to talk to except Satan and his devils.

Clismar said *The Post* cliticism must be taken seriously. If Milungu wants to be the Chief Executive he will have no time for showing young nuns what is meant by sin, or for giving consolation to lonely young women.

So we all agreed that if Milungu wants the job, he must resign from being an archbishop, and confine his conjugal services to one wife. St Simon said that he himself had been faithful to the same woman for over fifty years, and that's why he had been made a saint.

Sunday

I clied with joy when I saw the wedding on CNN. All went so perfectly. The brave Archbishop just walked into the Moon Cash and Carry, and bought a bride off the shelf. She's a Sin Sang, made in Korea. She has a tellibly pale skin, so he got 20% off. She must have overdone the Ambi.

And the other good news is that the Pope excommunicated him straight away, for not marrying a nun. So he'll be back in Zambia soon, to save my littul Fleddie!

Monday

Oh *Dear Diary*! Everything went wrong at the airport! Milungu was arrested for attempting to avoid duty on Korean imports. Sin Sang was arrested for having a marriage certificate which had not been approved by the Ministry of Commerce.

I know Satan is behind all this! If only my darling Fleddie knew what was going on!

31st May 2001

Chapter 7
Third Term Madness

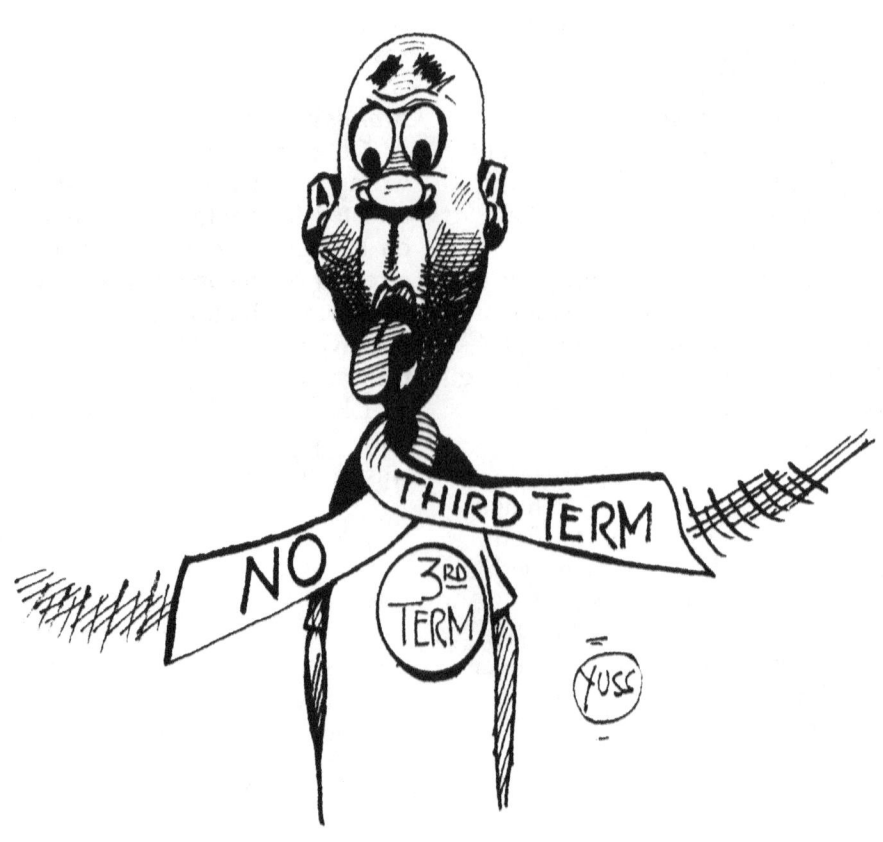

7.1 The Official Candidate

The President walked into the room and sat down at his polished desk. 'Good morning ladies and gentlemen. I am no longer your Official Candidate. I am now President Candidate!'

'Ha ha! Ho he!' everybody hooted 'What wit! How clever! What a genius!'

'Yes,' whispered Sam in my ear. 'When you get to be President, everything you say is very profound and witty.'

I looked at the date on my newspaper: 3rd November 2001. I felt dizzy. 'Where have I been the past year?' I hissed at Sam. 'I can't remember anything! What's happening?'

'Don't you worry about it.' said Sam, putting his arm round me. 'We've been looking after you. You're alright again now.'

'Who is this guy all wrapped up in bandages?'

'Its our new President,' whispered Sam. 'This is his first press conference since being elected.'

'Having been elected as the Official Candidate,' began the President. *'it is my job to appoint all the other official candidates. Therefore I appoint Mr Munchilinganya Munchishanya as Speaker of the National Assembly.'*

'I thought,' I whispered to Sam, 'that the Speaker had to be elected by the MPs.'

'That's only a formality,' whispered Sam, 'because the MPs were all appointed by the Official Candidate, as his official candidates.'

'But I thought they had to be elected by their constituencies,' I said.

'That's only a formality,' whispered Sam. 'Everybody has to vote for their official candidate.'

'But what's his real name? And why's he covered all over in bandages?'

'Nobody knows who he is, or where he came from. That's why he's covered in bandages. His name is Official Candidate. That's all we know.'

'Some of you,' continued President Official Candidate, *'may not understand the workings of our democratic system, which was given to us by my glorious predecessor, the father of democracy, Frederick Chiluba.*

'Frederick Chiluba provided the foundation of our democracy, because he was democratically elected. Therefore all democracy comes from him. So when he appointed me as his Official Candidate, democracy was legitimately passed on to me. Having been democratically appointed, it followed automatically that I was democratically elected.'

This provoked the party faithful into an ecstatic chant,

Our Father he gave us,
Our Candidate, our Leader!
One Party, one Candidate!
One Candidate, one Leader!
That leader, our President!

'Having been democratically elected,' continued the President, 'it is therefore my democratic duty to appoint all other official candidates, so that they can be democratically elected in the same way. This was all explained to us by the Founding Father of Democracy, our Great Teacher, Frederick Chiluba.

'I still don't understand.' I said, as we came out of the press conference, 'why he is all wrapped up in bandages.'

'Its quite simple really,' said Sam. 'Everybody pledged to vote for the Official Candidate before his identity was announced, merely because he was the choice of our Founding Father.'

'So his identity didn't matter?'

'Exactly,' said Sam. 'It was soon realised that it would be much better if he remained without any identity. If he was from the North, he would lose votes in the South, and vice versa. So, in his great wisdom, our Founding Father saw that without identity, the Official Candidate could rise above all tribal and regional considerations.'

'He might have a criminal record,' I suggested.

'Doesn't matter. People voted for him purely because he was the Official Candidate, which was above mere personal considerations. If his identity had been revealed, then people would have wanted to vote according to his abilities and record. That would have been quite wrong.'

'Quite wrong?'

'You've been away for over a year,' laughed Sam, 'you're a bit out of touch. Elections based on personalities lead to all sorts of mud-slinging. The peace of our country could have been threatened. There might have been anarchy. But you can't criticise a person if you don't know who he is!'

'Maybe Jesus has come back.' I suggested.

'Many believe so,' said Sam. 'After all, we're a Christian Nation.'

'Half a minute,' I said, 'What about his parentage? He'd be disqualified if he had an Israeli mother.'

'If you don't have any identity, laughed Sam. 'then nobody can prove that your parents weren't born in Zambia.'

'Even so,' I said, 'It still looks a bit weird to me. Suppose this Official Candidate is still being controlled by the previous president? By the way, where is he?'

'That's the funny thing,' said Sam. 'He disappeared the same day that he introduced his Official Candidate!'

6th April 2000

7.2 False Pretences

PRESIDENT Kadoli was waiting to begin the Cabinet meeting. He was lolling back on his cushions, with his feet up on the table, and his eyes staring inscrutably at the ceiling. At the other end of the table sat old Cycle Mata, his bloodshot eyes scowling at his Cabinet papers, as his blackened and broken teeth chewed upon an evil smelling cigar.

'So let's start the meeting,' said Kadoli, his eyes still heavenward, as if talking to God. 'Do we have the minutes of the previous meeting? When was that?'

'3rd December 1997,' chuckled old Cycle Mata, brushing the cigar ash from a yellowed piece of paper.

'And have we approved the minutes?' asked Kadoli.

'Unanimously,' declared the old ruffian.

'So what's the first item on today's agenda?'

'There's only one item on the agenda, Mr President,' declared Cycle Mata. 'I am putting a motion before the meeting that *the Cabinet agrees with all decisions of the President.*'

'Very good,' laughed Kadoli, still talking to the ceiling. 'Both God and myself demand absolute loyalty. If my ministers can't agree to a straightforward motion like that, obviously they must be plotting against me. Let me hear first from my Minister for Property.'

'Mr Sorry Mulenga is not here, Mr President, and sends his apologies. He's just been arrested on suspicion of obtaining money from a bank by false pretences.'

'A very sorry situation! If he wants to get money honestly, he should ask God. If he wants to get money by false pretences, he should ask parliament. OK, let's hear from some of the others. What about a quick quack from Quack Quackwi? She always has a quack on every subject, just like a man.'

'That's the problem, Mr President. I have sent her down to South Africa for medical tests and sexual classification. She may have joined the Cabinet under false pretences.'

'But doesn't Quack Quakwi have a boyfriend?' asked Kadoli, leaning back on his cushions, and blowing another halo of smoke towards God.

'That only makes it worse. They should both be in prison!'

'I thought she'd just returned from maternity leave?'

'She got it under false pretences. Under Party Rule 577, sub-section 1034, it is an offence for a man to claim maternity leave. Therefore Quack Quackwi has been expelled from the party.'

'What about the Minister of Illegal Affairs?' said Kadoli, now scowling angrily at the ceiling, 'what does he have to say on the subject?'

'He's out of town, investigating a judge who obtained six government houses by false pretences!'

'What false pretences?'

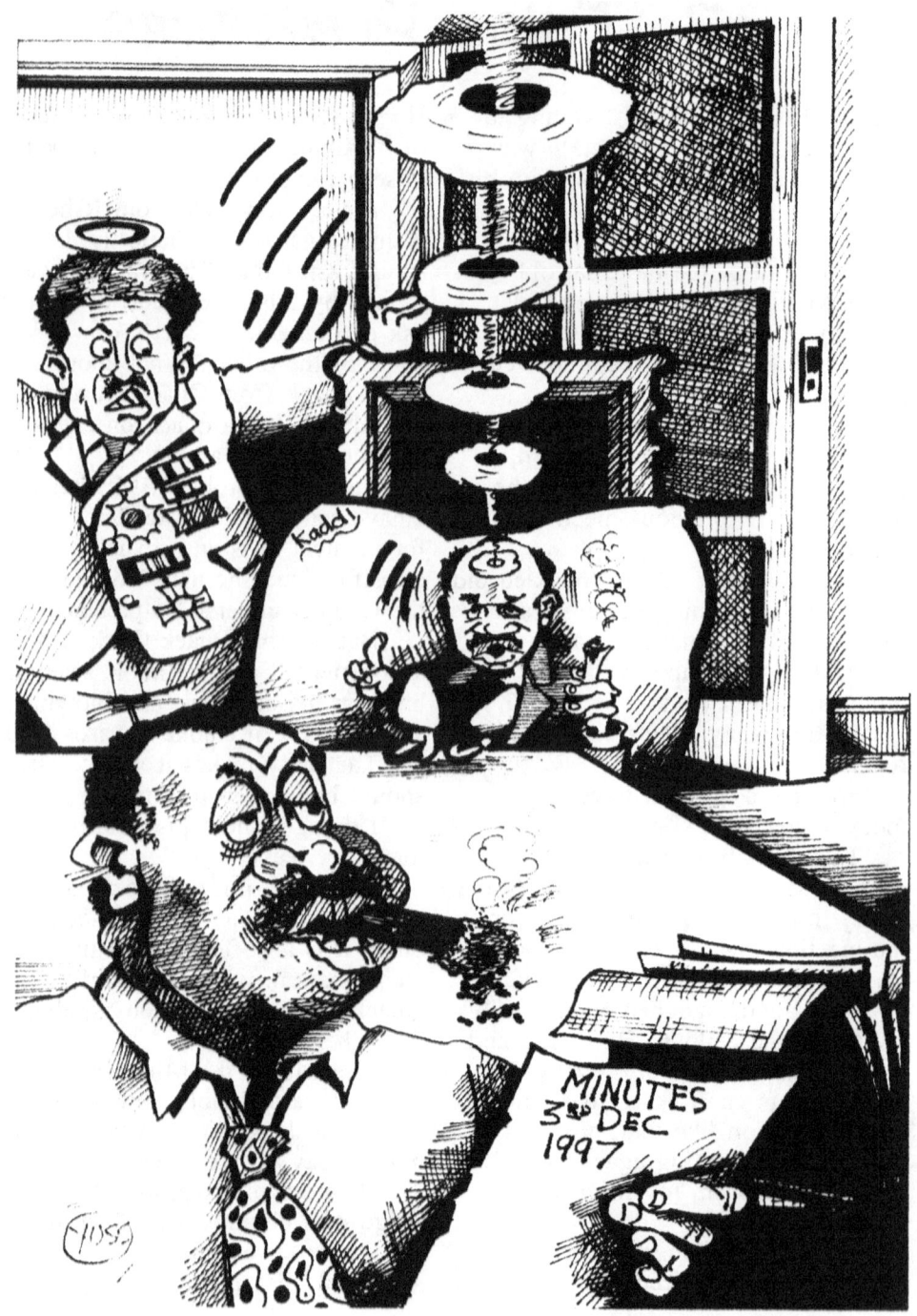

'It was claimed that the judge was growing so fat that a sixth house had become necessary to accommodate the accumulating folds of flesh.'

Kadoli leaned back further on his chair, and closed his eyes completely. 'Then let me hear from my Minister for Misinformation.'

'He's being questioned by the Anti Curriculum Committee, under suspicion of obtaining a certificate by false pretences.'

'Probably got it from Blantyre Market,' chuckled Kadoli, amidst another puff of smoke.

'And what about the Minister for Ethnic Minorities?'

'He's been deported, after it was discovered that one of his sixteen great great grandparents was born in Bombay. Apparently he obtained his passport by false pretences.'

'Then what is the opinion of the Minister for Agricultural Policy?'

'We've never had an Agricultural Policy!'

'Of course, I must have been dreaming!' Suddenly he sat up straight, opened his eyes, and looked down the table. 'My God! Where is everybody! There's nobody here except you and me! Where are all the others? Is this disloyalty, or just unpunctuality?'

'Hard to say,' laughed the old ruffian. 'Unpunctuality can be a sign of disloyalty, or maybe just diarrhoea.'

'At least all my loyal chairs are still here,' said Kadoli.

Just then the door burst open, and in stormed the Minister for Changing Principles, General Godless Meander.

'Are you a man or a woman?' asked Kadoli.

'What are you two doing here?' shouted the General. 'Weren't you told about the change of venue? I've just come from the Cabinet Meeting at the Oasis Restaurant! You've both been impeached for collecting votes under false pretences!'

'What!' screamed Kadoli, as he fell off his cushions and hit the floor with a thud. 'That's a lie! Nobody ever voted for me! They just voted against the other fellow!'

But old Cycle Mata just sat impassively in his seat, 'Under the constitution,' he growled, 'your impeachment motion is completely invalid.'

'How's that?' asked the General.

'In your absence,' declared Cycle Mata, 'this meeting has unanimously agreed to amend the constitution. False pretences have now been legalised!'

5th April 2001

7.3 Hippomania

'DID you read that article about Zambia in the *New African* last month?' asked Sara.

'Which one was that?' I asked.

'The one by Regina Mfubu. She had just returned to Zambia after being absent for ten years, and found the place to be much better than when she left!'

'Then she must be a hippopotamus!' I laughed.

'You've really got uncanny intuition,' laughed Sara. 'She is a hippopotamus! In her article she wrote how Zambia is now a much better place for hippos. Ten years ago there were nine million people and only one million hippos. Now there are only five million people, but six million hippos!'

'And all doing well!' I laughed.

'Oh yes,' said Sara. 'Hippos don't need clinics, or fees to send their children to school, They just need plenty of water and grass. They're not affected by the crisis in the balance of payments, or the falling kwacha. They are the only ones who have done really well under the government's economic policy.'

'They must have been very grateful when the government opened the Kariba Dam gates, and flooded all Chiawa. The hippos ate all the farmers' maize!'

'That's right,' said Sara. 'And they have benefited from government policy on protecting wildlife. The people have died, but the hippos have multiplied.'

'Perhaps,' I suggested, 'its the hippos who are behind this campaign for a Third Term.'

'Let's turn on the news,' laughed Sara, 'and see if you're right.'

The face of Evelyn Mutuntushi filled the TV screen. *'At a provincial party conference in Luangwa this morning, the Minister without Shame, Mr Recycled Salaula, addressed party cadres on the importance of democracy.'*

The screen now filled with the face of crafty old Salaula. 'My God,' said Sara, 'I didn't realise his face was so large. And look at those teeth!'

'Perhaps he's turning into a hippo,' I said.

'Democracy,' began Salaula, *'means that we must listen to everybody's opinion. As you know, the majority of the population here in Luangwa are hippos, who are solidly behind the government, and in favour of the Third Term. We in the party do not discriminate against hippos, provided both their parents are born in Zambia.*

'Some people say,' continued Salaula, *'that hippos have small brains, because they always used to vote for Old Munshumfwa and the One Party State. But democracy is about counting heads, not the content of heads. Hippos also have their opinion, and their opinion carries weight. I call upon you all to join the hippos, and put your weight behind the Third Term.'*

'It looks as if he's already joined the hippos,' said Sara, 'look at the way his face is swelling. Look at those jowls and bulging eyes. Look at the others on the platform! They're all turning into hippos! That must be the reason why the human population is decreasing, but hippos are increasing!'

The news reader Evelyn Mutuntushi returned to our screen. 'Look at the size of her!' shouted Sara. 'She'll break that little chair! She's turning into one as well!'

'In a separate development,' said Evelyn Hippo, *'the Minister for Cosmetic Change, Nkanda Blue, has ordered that all those supporting the Third Term should identify themselves by painting themselves in the party colour, blue.'*

'Look at her,' laughed Sara. 'She looks like a blue hippo.'

'Don't exaggerate,' I said, 'its just that she's overdone the eye makeup.'

'In a political demonstration this afternoon,' continued Evelyn Hippo, *'the party faithful marched on Parliament to demand a change in the Constitution.'*

The film clip showed an enormous crowd of blue monsters slowly converging on Manda Hill.

'That's an easy way to demonstrate,' I laughed. 'They've hired minibuses.'

'They're not minibuses,' said Sara pointing at the fuzzy picture on our old TV. 'Look more closely! They're blue hippos! Everybody has turned into a hippo! They're being led by Sorry Mulenga, who's also turned into a hippo.'

'He's always looked like that,' I said. 'But what are the police doing? Looks like they've set up a road-block!'

'They're arresting all the hippos which are not painted blue!' laughed Sara.

'They can't let disloyal party members into parliament!'

'In a late news item just arrived,' announced Evelyn Hippo, *'a stampede of hippos has just invaded parliament demanding a Third Term. They have razed the National Assembly Building to the ground and eaten all the documents, including all the laws and the Constitution.'*

'My God,' I said. 'They've destroyed Democracy and the Constitution!'

'Not destroyed,' laughed Sara. 'Only eaten. What goes in one end has to come out the other!'

'You're right,' I said. 'What comes out will make a firm foundation for the Third Term.'

25th January 2001

7.4 Gospel Truth

I was dozing on the back pew of St Ignominious when Sara gave me a sharp elbow in the ribs. 'Wake up! Father Joe Kombokombo is going to read the lesson!'

'He keeps reading from the same book,' I growled.

But I sat up straight to listen to the famous cleric when he began reading from the Gospel according to St Kalaki, Chapter 23, verses 1-16...

Then the Chief Thug of Jerusalem, the Mighty Shatta, gathered together all his bakaponya, and took Jesus before the judge Pompous Pilot, accusing him of heresy and blasphemy, and savouring sausage on the Sabbath.

And Pompous Pilot spoke unto Jesus, saying 'You are accused of calling yourself Jesus Constitution, as if all laws and rules come from you. Is this true?'

And Jesus answered him, saying 'Its because I am the Constitution that I have no place in this court, for I am the one who governs this court, and all other courts. I am the truth and the word and the light. It is not for some little kaponya dressed up as a judge to be asking me such impertinent questions. Rather it is for me to question your behaviour.'

'See how he insults you!' crowed the Chief Thug, 'He imagines he is above us, and can lay down the law. But I say unto him that it is we who are supposed to be in charge of the Constitution, not the Constitution in charge of us! This awkward Constitution thinks he is a man, but he is just a piece of paper. And like a piece of paper, we shall nail him to the cross!'

'Yebo!' shouted the crowd of bakaponya, waving their pangas and knobkerries. 'Teach him a lesson! Crucify him! Crucify him!'

'For a fair debate we must hear both sides of this story,' said Pilot. 'You, Jesus that call yourself the Constitution, what do you have to say for yourself?'

'Your question is mistaken, for the Constitution cannot defend itself. It has to be defended by others. It has to be defended by wisdom, morality, legality and truth.'

'Crucify them all!' chanted the crowd.

'However, I should point out,' said Jesus, speaking quietly above the cacophony, 'that I am defended by all the lawyers and attorneys in the land.'

'They are just a small minority of the population,' shouted the Chief Thug. 'It is we thieves and liars who are in the majority!'

'Majority rules!' shouted the crowd.

'In addition,' continued Jesus calmly, 'I am defended by all the worshippers in all the synagogues.'

'We have excommunicated them all,' announced the Chief Thug, as the crowd fell about laughing.

'And I am also defended by ministers of the government.'

'They were all fired last week,' chortled the Chief Thug, 'I am just about to send them a backdated letter.'

'And most of all,' Jesus continued calmly through the cheering and jeering, 'I am defended by the truth. Whoever belongs to the truth listens to me.'

'Truth is merely in the head,' scoffed the Chief Thug. 'It can be sliced off with a panga.'

Now Pompous Pilot turned to the crowd of liars, pickpockets and thugs, and said unto them, 'What do you want me to do with this man?'

'Crucify him! Crucify him!' they shouted.

'This is the Feast of the Passover,' said Pompous Pilot, 'when the nation traditionally passes over from reason into madness, and from order into chaos. In order to aggravate the general lunacy, I always release a prisoner at this time of year.'

'Don't release him! Crucify him, crucify him!'

'But it was only yesterday,' said Pompous Pilot, 'that another crowd told me to crucify the Great Thief Wabufi, for stealing the people's taxes. Now whom should I release? Which one should I crucify? Wabufi or the Constitution?'

'Release Wabufi!' chanted the thieves. 'He is one of us! Give us Wabufi, and crucify the Constitution!'

'Since the Roman Empire is famous all over the world as a democracy,' said Pompous Pilot, 'I shall follow the will of the people. Therefore, I give your Wabufi back to you, and this Jesus Constitution shall be crucified!'

And so saying, Pompous Pilot climbed up on his bench and tore off his judge's wig and gown, and revealed his true self to the crowd. 'It is I, the Great Wabufi!'

'Another great performance!' applauded the crowd. 'The Great Wabufi is back! Thief amongst thieves! Joker amongst jokers! Judge in his own case! Now he has crucified the Constitution, he can rule for evermore!'

'Here endeth the First Lesson,' declared Father Kombokombo.

'Powerful stuff!' I whispered to Sara. 'I wonder what happened to Israel after that?'

'Civil war,' said Sara, 'which has continued even to this very day.'

'And now,' said Father Kombokombo in sombre tone and trembling voice, 'Let us pray.'

15th March 2001

7.5 Ratification

THE TV news had just finished and Sara was still laughing. 'When real life is so ridiculous,' she cackled, 'you're wasting your time trying to write comedy.'

'There's a thin line between comedy and tragedy,' I said.

'And Manasseh Phiri is just about to cross it,' sniggered Sara, as the deadly *Health Matters* hit the screen like a lump of cold porridge.

'In addition to the epidemics of AIDS, cholera and TB,' began Manasseh, 'we now have to struggle with the new outbreak of Kafupi Plague.'

'Yes,' sighed Sara, 'this government will be remembered for the many things it brought to the people.'

'Kafupi Plague,' continued Manasseh, 'is caused by a little parasite ...'

'That originated in Ndola,' cackled Sara.

'That originated in Zaire,' said Manasseh.

'He might be right' laughed Sara.

'This little parasite is carried by a type of termite,' explained Manasseh, 'which goes through a life cycle of three terms. In its first term it lives simply in the soil, as the little inswa we all know and love. But in its second term it invades the bodies of rats!'

'Or politicians!' suggested Sara.

'The termite's third term, sometimes called the terminator, comes when there is a great flood, or a huge slush fund, and the rats can spread everywhere. Particularly when there is a sinking ship, the rats have to swim for it, and the termites go looking for another host. This is the stage when they can enter human flesh.'

'Of the Third Termers,' said Sara.

'We shouldn't blame the humble little termite for the Plague any more than we should blame the mosquito for malaria,' said Manasseh. 'The Plague is actually carried by the little Kafupi virus, which the poor termite picks up from the rat, and then passes on to humans. Once this greedy little Kafupi virus has entered the bloodstream, it gradually turns the human brain into the brain of a rat. It is estimated that ten percent of the entire population is now infected with the Kafupi virus.'

'The politicians,' laughed Sara. 'They're the ones who are getting infected. They're all slowly turning into Third Termers.'

'This is no laughing matter,' I said. 'This could infect the whole nation. We could all turn into rats!'

'I am now sitting in the office of a once famous politician,' said Manasseh, 'who is showing symptoms of the disease.'

He certainly didn't look well. His eyes were staring vacantly at the ceiling, saliva drooled from his gaping mouth, and his blackened teeth snarled at the camera.

Manasseh put his hand gently on

the poor fellow's shoulder. 'How do you explain your present condition?'

He tried to find a few words to explain himself, but succeeded only in producing a drunken belch.

'What a ghastly sight,' said Sara. 'No wonder his wife left him.'

'Apart from his deteriorating physical condition,' said Manasseh, 'the Kafupi virus has completely corrupted his moral sense, leading to unbridled and ungovernable greed. Altruism has given way to selfishness. Honour to dishonour. Loyalty has turned to treachery. Just as his appearance has become abject and shabby, so his behaviour has become malicious, degenerate and contemptible. The parasite has destroyed his constitution, just as he will now destroy the constitutions of others. As a result of this corruption, all his promises have been broken, and all his directions and values have been reversed.'

Manasseh now turned to the pathetic victim, and spoke gently to him. 'When I say a word, see if you can think of a similar word. Let's start with the word Democracy.'

'Ratocracy,' snapped the patient.

'Power?' asked Manasseh.

'Thug,' said the rat.

'Vote?' suggested Manasseh.

'Bribe,' replied the rat.

'Unity?'

'Tribe,' retorted the rat.

'Nation?'

'Race,' laughed the rat.

'Constitution?'

'Just paper,' squealed the rat. 'We rats eat paper!'

'Human rights?'

'Ratification!'

'Come on Manasseh,' I said to the TV, 'now tell us how to cure it! Can we just boil our drinking water?'

'Or boil the rats,' suggested Sara.

'Now you may be wondering,' said Manasseh, again addressing the viewers, 'how to protect yourself from this terrible disease. All you have to do is to cut a piece of green ribbon, and ...'

Just then there was a terrible squealing noise as a monster rat came bounding into our sitting room, with the cat chasing after it.

'Aaargh ...Aaargh ...!' I screamed, as I went rigid with fear, and Sara jumped onto the sofa.

'Don't be frightened, Grandpa,' laughed Katendi, as she pulled off her mask. 'What a silly Grandpa you are! It was only a joke!'

'Katendi,' I said, as I managed to regain control of myself, 'there are some things we shouldn't joke about!'

29th March 2001

7.6 Rising to the Occasion

BENNY Sinn was lying in his white silk dressing gown by the poolside of his mansion in California, eating a breakfast of prawns and champagne, and reading his morning mail. By his side sat the luscious Baby Doll, brushing her long blonde hair, as the sun shone straight through her transparent negligee, revealing all her excellent qualifications.

'Listen to this,' sniggered Sinn, reading from the letter he was holding, 'Oh Heavenly Messenger and Miracle Worker ...'

'Hmmmm,' murmured Baby Doll softly, as she nibbled his ear, 'you certainly were heavenly last night.'

'It's a letter from Africa,' laughed Sinn, taking another gulp of champagne, as Baby Doll curled around him.

'Is that in California?' purred Baby Doll, as she explored the inside of his ear with her tongue.

'Its some awful American colony,' said Sinn, 'somewhere east of Florida. That's where I made my money, amongst the gullible natives, doing circus crusades and other supernatural entertainment for Sunshine Miracles Incorporated. Easy money, we collected millions. That's how I managed to move to California, and set up Sunshine Sexual Services.'

'You certainly are a miracle,' she cadoodled, slipping her hand inside his dressing gown. 'Give me a little taste of Sinn for breakfast.'

'Its from one of their Presidents,' said Sinn, still managing to concentrate on the letter, 'who apparently still believes I am a prophet and messenger from God.'

'I can feel another miracle coming up, darling,' drooled Baby Doll.

'You can send me to heaven right now if you like. Tell me about what he says, you've really got my juices going.'

'Stop titillating me, you naughty girl,' tittered Sinful Sinn, as he began to read from the letter.

'Oh Saintly Sinn, please pray for me and my presidency, for I am surrounded by pagans and infidels who refuse to believe I am appointed by God to rule this land.'

'I'll get all the girls to bend down in prayer tonight,' giggled Baby Doll, 'that always gets the bishop excited!'

'The pagans and infidels are now saying,' continued Sinn, reading the letter, 'that I was elected by them, not appointed by God. And the Christians have been holding services all over the land, asking God to appoint somebody else.

'You were the one, O Sanctified Sinn, who told me I was appointed by God. I have been on my knees every night, asking God to verify the information, but I have received no answer.'

'I always like a man on his knees,' laughed Baby Doll, 'when I give him holy communion.'

'Oh my most Sublime and Spiritual Sinn, can you please contact the Lord and ask Him whether my contract has been extended, or if I can please go to heaven now, because right now I'm in a hell of a mess.'

'Archbishop Swaggering Swaggert's coming tonight,' giggled Baby Doll, 'to give delicious penance and holy communion to Busty Barbara. Perhaps he could have a word with God before he gets too exhausted.'

'Please my Miracle Messenger, have another word with God, and check on my appointment, because He's not listening to me. And all the lawyers have deserted me, claiming that I was holding the Holy Bible when I swore to defend the Constitution. They're lying. I was holding a copy of The Prince by Machiavelli, which I happened to be reading at the time.

'Even the trade unions have declared war against me, and my own cabinet is laughing in my face. I am supported by only six headmen from Kasama, one of whom is blind and deaf. Even my wife has left me. I am all alone. Please help O Sanctimonious and Supernatural Sinn.'

'The poor man is terribly depressed,' said Baby Doll. 'Perhaps we could send him Sexy Sandra for a couple of nights. That might get his pecker to perk up! Come on you naughty prophet and miracle worker! What are you going to do for him?'

Then the Great Sinn stood up straight and took a white hood out of his pocket, and put it over his head. He stuck out his arm in a Nazi salute and cast his words boldly to the wind. 'Plant the fiery crosses across the land and burn the homes of the pagans and infidels! I am the Messenger of the Lord! I am the Grand Wizard of the Ku Klux Klan, appointed to defend the word of the Lord against all traitors, foreigners, blacks, adulterers, abortionists, foreigners, homosexuals, communists, witches, sorcerers, hooters, honkers, whistlers and especially people from Bombay. The Lord's Messenger must be respected!'

'Oooh,' said Baby Doll, throwing her arms around him, and pressing herself against him, 'I love a man who can rise to the occasion!'

12th April 2001

7.7 Follow the Rules

LAST Sunday morning Sara and I had just sat down to a late breakfast when swinging in through the front door came a pair of tight blue jeans, balanced precariously on a massive pair of platform boots. Our daughter Namukolo was back from boarding school.

'So how was Chisamba Girls?' I asked, as she greeted us. 'Did you manage to settle down and do some work?'

'Hah!' she cackled. 'I can't go back there! That place is finished!'

'It was running very well when we took you there,' said Sara sternly. 'Are you the one responsible?'

'Funny you should ask that,' laughed Namukolo, as she took a sip of tea, her metallic blue finger nails glinting in the morning sun. 'It was my history project that started all the trouble.'

'I don't know how you do it,' said Sara. 'You burnt down St Marys with your cookery project.'

'You've always been against me,' snapped Namukolo.

'Don't start all that again,' Sara retorted. 'Just tell us what happened.'

'For my project, I decided to write a history of the school. So I spent every afternoon in the school library, delving into the records.'

'There's a school library?' I laughed. 'It must be the last one in the country!'

'Well, actually its just some boxes of old yellow papers, stored under the stage. It was terrible under there, with the cockroaches and rats. Half of the papers had been eaten by the rats. But what I found shook the foundations of the school!'

'Did you find the corpse of the previous headmaster?'

'Worse than that, I found the CV of the present headmaster!'

'Not qualified?'

'Worse than that! Born in 1945! Fifty-six years old!'

'What's wrong with that?'

'He's past his shelf life! You see, I also found the original School Rules, written by the White Sisters in 1927, which state that all teachers must retire at fifty-five.'

'So what did you do about it?'

'I put a motion before the School Debating Society that the Head must retire, since he is the very one who is always lecturing us about following the rules.'

'And what happened?'

'The meeting was broken up by the school prefects.'

'Sent by the headmaster?'

'He didn't have to. By protecting the appointing authority, they were protecting their privilege to eat all the meat, leaving the rest of us with rotten beans. Where do you think corruption comes from? It's taught in school! Don't you know anything!'

'There's no need to be cheeky,' Sara snapped.

'Perhaps I should be more polite by avoiding the truth,' sneered Namukolo.

'So what about the Head? I asked

quickly. 'Did he discipline the prefects?'

'Not at all,' laughed Namukolo. 'He said everybody should debate this very important question, but we should just be careful not to get whipped by prefects while doing so.'

'What about the teachers?' I asked. 'Didn't they support the School Rules?'

'Hah!' cackled Namukolo. 'Only those who thought they could get the top job, they were very much in favour of the School Rules!'

'And the others?'

'The other half were holders of forged or ungraded certificates, whose jobs were in the pocket of the Head. They were the ones who said never mind the rules, we should respect the Head, who has great vision.'

'And does he have great vision?'

'He has little squinty eyes, and wears dark glasses.'

'So were you able to prepare for your Form Five exams?' asked Sara.

'You must be joking,' laughed Namukolo. 'We spent every day in the school hall, with one side arguing for, and the other arguing against. Finally we all agreed to put the matter to a vote.

'The Head declared that according to the rules, the whole school community would vote. We would all stand in the school hall. Those in favour of changing the School Rule would go out through the side doors leading onto the playing field. Those against would remain in the hall.'

'So who won?'

'As soon as the Head shouted *Vote*, the prefects opened the doors under the stage, and chased out all the cockroaches and rats, through the doors and onto the playing field.'

'*I declare the rule changed by a huge majority* declared the Head.

'*Hey,* we shouted, *cockroaches can't vote!*'

'*According to Clause 99f of the School Rules,* declared the Head, *it clearly states that all members of the school community must have the vote!*

'*But cockroaches can't think,* we shouted.

'*In a democratic system,* declared the Head, *its only numbers that count.*'

'So what did you do then?' I asked.

'After that,' laughed Namukolo, 'we decided to reduce the number of cockroaches. So we burnt down the school.'

26th April 2001

7.8 The Presidential Candidate
Advertisement in The Daily Sellout 15th May 2001

Spectator Kalaki's Employment Agency on behalf of the Movement for Murdering Democracy

Advertisement for Presidential Candidate

Due to confusion at the recent Party Convention, the Movement for Murdering Democracy accidentally omitted to elect a Presidential Candidate. Applications are therefore invited from members of MMD who wish to put their names forward for consideration as the Presidential Candidate in the coming Republican Presidential Election.

Job Description

The Presidential Candidate will report directly to the Party President. The Candidate will follow all instructions given to him by the Party President, read all speeches officially given to him, and refer all questions to the Party President.

Using the Police Force and ZNBC as his campaign staff, the Candidate is expected to ensure his own unopposed election as Republican President. Thereafter he will be appointed Senior Ambassador to the Party President. He will represent his country abroad, while the Party President runs the country at home.

Whilst abroad, he will have special responsibilities for selecting suits and shoes for the Party President.

Previous Experience

It would be an advantage if the applicant has previous experience in:

- *Collecting bus fares;*
- *Twisting arms;*
- *Licking boots;*
- *Distributing brown paper envelopes;*
- *Doctoring lists of delegates;*
- *Mobilising multiple voting;*
- *Stuffing ballot boxes;*
- *Spoiling ballot papers;*
- *Organising countless recounts;*
- *Reinterpreting constitutions.*

Qualifications

Academic qualifications are not required, or even desirable. The successful applicant will be fitted up with appropriate certificates after the appointment. However, the successful applicant must be:

- *Fluent in Bemba;*
- *Fond of fancy suits;*
- *Able to dance to any tune.*

Long fingers would be an added advantage.

Personal Qualities

Rather than ability, the essential quality of the successful candidate will be self-confidence. In particular, it is expected that he will be able to:

- Look straight into the camera whilst lying;
- Say one thing whilst doing another;
- Demand loyalty from the blind;
- Praise all UN Conventions;
- Ignore human rights.

Claiming to be a Christian would be an added advantage.

Terms and Conditions of Service

The successful applicant will be given a five year contract, with prospect of renewal for a further five year term. There is no provision for a third term, so preference will be given to applicants who are unable to count up to three. However, the appointment may be terminated at any time, at the discretion of the Party President.

Once the Candidate has been installed as Republican President, accommodation will be provided at a small hotel in Paris. From there, he will be well placed to purchase suits for the Party President. Should he find it necessary to return home, temporary accommodation will be provided in the Servants Quarters of the Party President, at State House.

Remuneration will be in accordance with normal Civil Service salary scales, and commensurate with the scale for a District Administrator. Payment will be made quarterly, by brown paper envelope.

Selection Process

The Presidential Candidate will be selected by the Party President, at his sole discretion. However, according to the Party Constitution, the appointment has to be ratified by the next Party Convention, scheduled to take place in November 2011.

Method of Application

Letters of application should be sent to:

Cycle Mata
Brown Envelopes Division
MMD

Inclusion of a well stuffed brown paper envelope would be an added advantage.

Note: In line with Indigenous Policy, MMD is an unequal opportunity employer. Applicants of Asian descent should first go by foot to India, and then post their applications from Calcutta. Similarly, female applicants should first go by foot to the Women's Lobby, and then post their applications to:

Fester Nakawalala
Sewage Pond
Garden Compound

Chapter 8
Elections and Erections

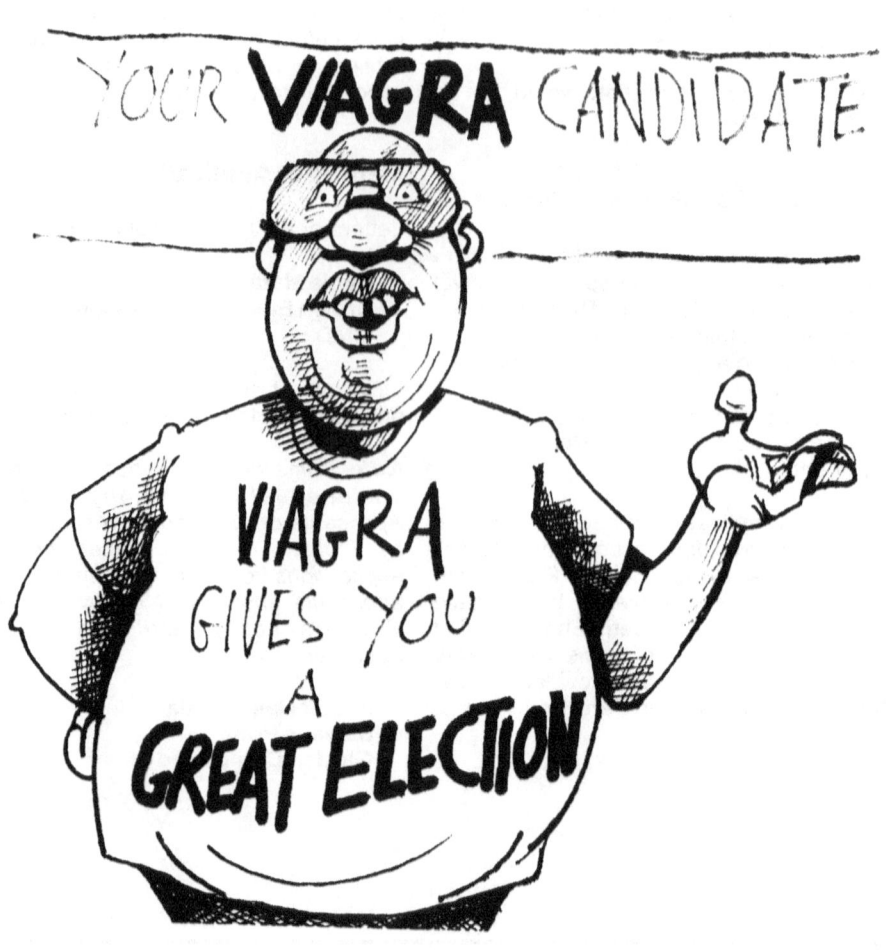

8.1 Road to Manda Hill

IT was three o'clock in the afternoon, but nothing of much interest had come down the wire from Reuters, and we had drawn a blank on the Internet. 'If Sir Fred comes in and finds we haven't got a story,' said Sam, 'he's going to get a bit ratty.'

'Let me show you the new Manda Hill,' said Sam. 'There's always something going on there. If not, we could easily provoke something.'

So off we footed, up the Great East. As we came to the traffic lights, there loomed into view a massive monstrosity, without shape or form, let alone architecture.

'My God,' I said. 'What's that? Another Namboard Depot? An aircraft hangar? Or has Simon Mwewa built himself another house?'

'Don't be silly,' laughed Sam. 'This is Manda Hill!'

'Who's being silly?' I snapped. 'There's no hill here at all. I thought we were heading for parliament.'

'This is where it all begins,' explained Sam. 'This is where you can buy all the things that will get you up the hill, and into parliament.'

As we got closer, I could see that the Manda Monstrosity was divided into different sections: *Political Game, Hoprite, Truthworth, Moore Flattery, Supreme Tarnishers,* and so on.

'Political Game is the most popular nowadays,' said Sam. 'Let's go in there.'

Each section had its own sign hanging from the ugly tin roof. *Nomination Game, Membership Game, Dark Corner Game, Expulsion Game,* and so on.

'Let's see what they've got in Electoral Game,' I said.

People were flocking around the shelves, where big notices advertised the goods on sale:

Forged membership cards, 1 gluder
Cards of deceased, 2 gluders
Cards of living, 3 gluders
Buy any two, get one free!
All National Party cards half Price!

'Now you can see,' said Sam, 'how the free market has liberated politics. Previously this was all done secretly up the Hill, and the rest of us didn't know what was going on. Now it's all come down the hill, where anybody with money can join in.'

'It's certainly come a long way down hill,' I admitted.

We walked on. Voter's Cards were going for only 10 gluders, and Voters Certificates for 15. But green reggies were priced at 50 gluders.

'Seems a bit steep,' I said. 'Down at the Green Registration Office, they come out the back door at only 20 gluders.'

'These are just the cheap things to give away to voters,' laughed Sam. 'But if you want to climb up the Hill, the expensive part is becoming indigenous.'

He pointed at the central display

of certificates in gold frames, with a big red notice saying

Genuine birth certificates while you wait! Only 500 gluders for a genuine indigenous parent. Buy one parent and get the other one free! You too can be President!

We walked down further to the Salaula Nikuv Computers, where a big sign read

Get your own Nikuv to ensure your own party members are on the Register. Special Delete Button to remove the opposition.

'All these things used to be secret,' explained Sam. 'But now we have transparency, so that everybody can see what's going on. Lets go and have a look at Hoprite. It's much more fun.'

'There aren't any commodities!' I exclaimed, as we walked in. 'Just people sitting on the shelves!'

'They are the commodities!' laughed Sam. 'Hoprite is where the party hoppers hop from one party to the next.'

On the shelf sat an ancient forlorn Munkombwe with a placard round his neck saying

Up and Down provincial chairman seeks job as Minister for Muddle in the Movement for Marketing Democracy.

The saliva dripped down his poor old chin as his left eye looked to the left, and his right eye to the right, trying to spot a prospective buyer.

'He can't get a job like that. For one thing, he's well past his shelf life. And for another,' said Sam, pointing to a chart on the wall, 'the exchange rate is well known.'

50 members = 1 district chair
10 district chairs = 1 prov. chair
10 prov. chairs = 1 MP
10 mps = 1 Minister

'But is that correct? I thought Independent MPs were supposed to be much more valuable than ordinary party MPs.'

'Its difficult to say,' replied Sam. 'There hasn't been enough trade to establish a firm market price.'

'But I heard that Chastity Mwansa was promised a job as Minister of Helicopters.'

'Yes, but up to now she hasn't been given anything,' laughed Sam. 'The silly girl made the mistake of trying to collect her own lobola! It's only her father who can be made Minister of Helicopters!'

'Before we go,' I said, 'let's have a look at Bookworld.'

'Actually, its called Cookworld. They sell specialised cookbooks and stationery.'

'How does that help you get up the Hill?'

'Winning an election is very similar to cooking a chicken. First you stuff the ballot box, then you cook the election!'

24th April 2000

8.2 The Silly Ass

LAST night Sara and I were watching the TVZ news, when suddenly the screen was filled with the smooth greasy ingratiating face of Mr Velvet Mango, Chief Liar of the Movement for Marketing Donkeys.

'Turn him off,' I pleaded. 'He gives me the creeps.'

'Its hard to believe,' laughed Sara, 'that this repellent creature is trying to attract votes. I'm fascinated.'

'It is my honour and privilege, as party spokesman,' began Velvet Mango, 'to report the result of our deliberations on the next Presidential Candidate. I'm sure the nation will fully appreciate the dilemma faced by our National Execution Committee, in that some of our best leaders have been executed, whilst others have fled the party, or even fled the country.'

'All that remains,' cackled Sara, 'are the snakes, hyenas and donkeys.'

'But we had to rid the party,' said Mango with a crafty leer, 'of these clever leaders, who misused their intelligence to manipulate the constitution, deceive the people and arrogate more power unto themselves. We are therefore of the considered opinion that the voters are now calling for a truly stupid leader, who is not suspected of having the brains to organise large scale theft and corruption.'

'Yes!' laughed Sara. 'Bring on the donkey!'

'It therefore gives me great pride and pleasure to present our new Presidential Candidate...'

So saying, he reached to his left, and pulled out an old grey donkey. 'I present to the nation Mr Eunuch Kapimpinya, a donkey with neither brains nor testicles. Completely harmless in all respects. A loveable leader at last!'

'*Hee-haw! Hee-haw!*' responded the donkey.

'God in his generosity and wisdom has given this Christian Nation a donkey to take us to the Promised Land, just as he gave Jesus a donkey to travel to Jerusalem.'

'Didn't that end in the crucifixion?' I asked.

'But are donkeys truly in-digenous?' wondered Sara. 'We don't want another foreigner on the throne.'

'Some people may ask,' leered Mango into the camera, his saliva dripping down the screen, 'whether a donkey is eligible to stand as a Presidential Candidate. It is my pleasure to allay any fears on this count. The party's legal advisor has assured us that, so long as both parents were born in Zambia, there is no bar to a donkey becoming President.'

'I can foresee one problem,' Sara said. 'I could get arrested for insulting the President if I called him a donkey. And suppose I called him a silly ass?'

'It can't be wrong to call him a donkey if he actually is a donkey,' I said. 'But according to the law you

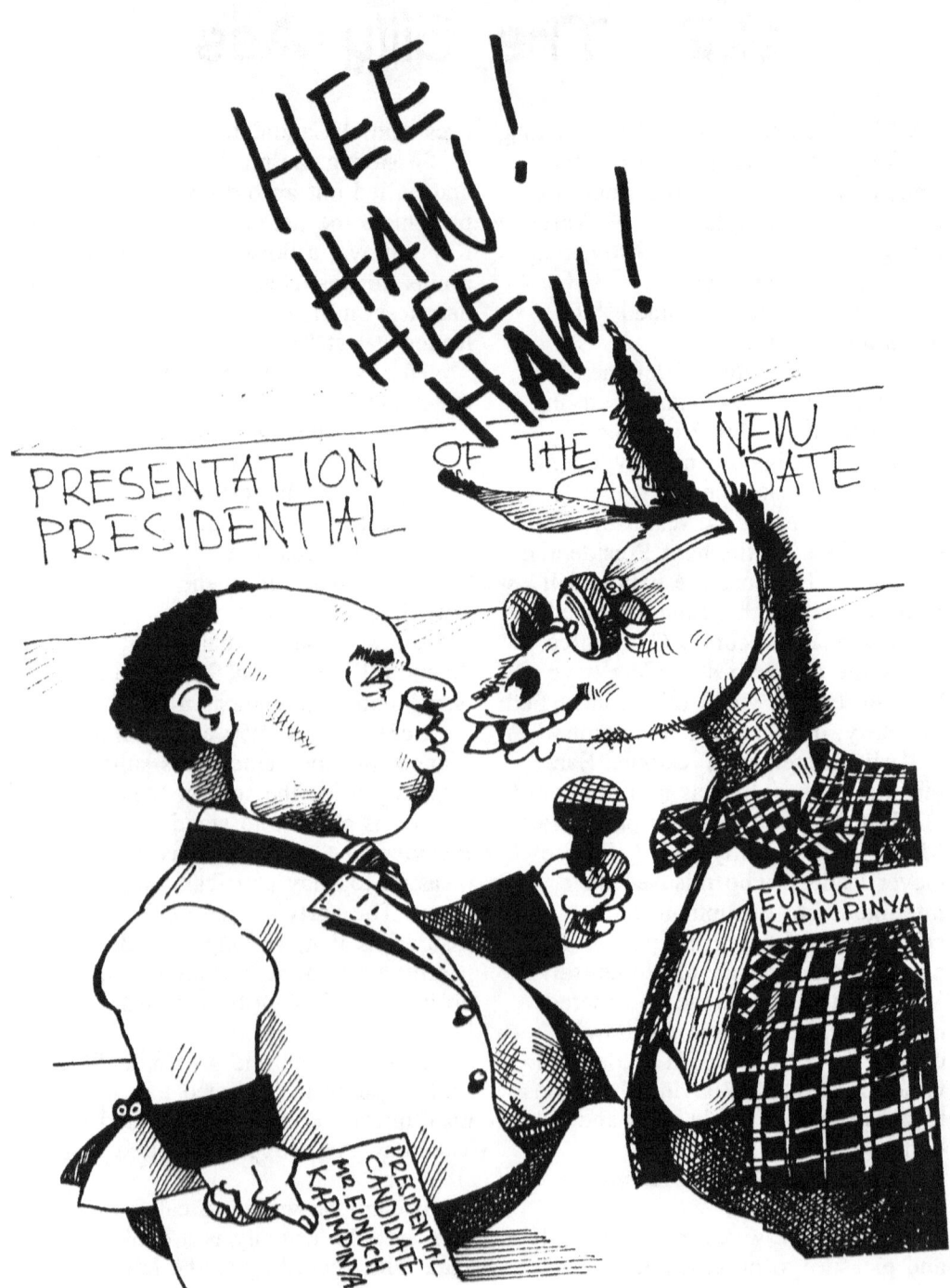

have to show respect to the Head of State. So it would be insulting to call him a silly ass, as if he were just an ordinary silly ass like other silly asses. You would have to refer to him as His Excellency the President Dr Silly Ass PhD. This is the form of politeness which is much appreciated by silly asses.'

As we were talking, the greasy Mango had lifted the donkey's foot onto the table. 'Look at this hoof!' he cried in triumph. 'Even if he had brains, how could he steal? Nobody can say he has long fingers! He doesn't have any fingers at all!'

'If the billions were loaded into a cart,' suggested Sara, 'he could pull them all the way from the National Assembly to State House.'

'Listen to the empty echo,' said Mango in triumph, as he rapped the donkey's skull with his knuckles. 'Absolutely nothing between the ears.'

'Maybe he's like most men,' said Sara, 'with his brains in his testicles.'

'It's a good thing he can't hear what you're saying,' I laughed.

Whereupon Mango turned the donkey round, and displayed its rear end to the camera. 'Most important of all, no testicles! No problem of this one producing spoilt brats to terrorise the nation!

'And no more wasting government funds on pomp and splendour. No need for a Mercedes, he'll be able to trot to all official functions. No need for State House banquets, he eats only grass. He'll feed off the State House lawns, and deposit his dung in the flowerbeds. He won't even need to occupy State House!'

'Of course not!' laughed Sara, 'because the present incumbent will be staying on!'

'Last of all,' cried Mango, turning again towards the donkey, 'I shall ask the donkey a few questions, so you can see how really stupid he is.

'What's the different between 40% and 100%?' asked Mango.

'Hee-haw' replied the donkey.

'What's the difference between a doctor and a nurse?'

'Hee-her,' laughed the donkey.

'What's the difference between a diamond and an AK47?'

'A *million dollars!*' retorted the donkey.

'He shouldn't have said that!' I exclaimed.

'But it does show,' laughed Sara, 'that he really is a silly ass!'

26th July 2001

8.3 Super Salesman

LAST Tuesday I decided to drop in on the famous Velvet Mango, the super salesman of the Movement for Marketing Dummies. I found him in his garden, watering his cabbages.

'Spectator Kalaki!' he said, walking towards me and extending his hand. 'I saw you on the TV last night! What are you up to? Are you beginning your presidential campaign?'

'Exactly,' I said. 'I thought, with all your experience, you could give me a few tips.'

'First of all,' he said, looking me up and down, 'you have to keep it zipped in front of the cameras.'

'Oops,' I said, looking down and adjusting my trousers. 'I certainly don't want to make other men jealous.'

'That was always my problem,' sighed Velvet, 'I always revealed too much of myself.' A tear rolled down his greasy oval face.

'Never mind,' I said, putting my arm around him. 'I think you're a delicious old Mango, and a super salesman. If you can sell me as a leader, it would be the crowning achievement of your extraordinary life.'

'It would indeed,' he said. 'Were your parents born in Zambia?'

'Both in UK.'

'What!' chortled Velvet. 'To have one parent born abroad may be taken as an unfortunate accident. But both of them, that's absolutely inexcusable! Don't you realise that becoming president takes a lot of forward planning! And you begin by having both your parents born in the wrong place! Very careless! What sort of president would you make?'

'I'm sorry,' I said. 'My mind must have been somewhere else at the time. So what do we do now?'

'Don't worry,' he said. 'This is where my Movement for Marketing Dummies comes in. We shall find a dummy to stand in for you, as your presidential candidate. Of course you can remain in charge. What are you calling your party?'

'Dunno. How about the Marvellous Musungu Democracy?'

'Splendid,' laughed Velvet. 'People are fed up with the Mad Muntu Dictatorship. They're in the mood for change!'

'So where shall we find the dummy?'

'That's what I'm doing right now. I'm preparing the ground for new leaders.'

'All I can see is cabbages.'

'Exactly. We have always said that a hungry man cannot talk of democracy. People are fed up with nothing but talk and no food. They are even refusing to vote for politicians. But they will vote for food. So we shall give them cabbage!'

'Somebody from the grassroots!'

'Exactly! We shall call your new leader the Great Cabbage, the

Mwansabamba Kabeji. The man who grew up in the grassroots, who believes development should be bottom-up!'

'Not up-bottom!'

'There's been too much up-bottom, due to the corruption of morals by TV. Now we need a leader with real roots in the Zambian soil. This will pull the people together, united around one ideological principle, one concept of leadership, one national destiny, one culture, all symbolised by the Mighty Cabbage...

*One Nation, One Cabbage,
One Cabbage, One Leader!*

'Its beginning to make sense,' I admitted. 'But what happens if the people become dissatisfied with their leader?'

'No problem!' laughed Velvet. 'They can eat him! Cabbages are easily replaceable! Instead of the leaders eating the people's money, let the people eat their leaders! This will further strengthen our democracy, as we move from bottom-up to bottom-down.'

'But perhaps the people themselves will begin to turn into cabbages!'

'That will stop the brain drain! Differentials of birth and wealth will disappear when we have achieved the equality of the cabbage! Both leaders and followers will have their feet planted firmly in the ground. All on the same footing! Equality and democracy at last!'

'But don't you have to give leadership training, before a cabbage can take its rightful place as president?'

'Of course,' laughed Mango, as his front gates swung upon, and a cavalcade of twenty four motor cycles and five Mercedes came swinging up the drive with sirens blaring *'Hee Haw! Hee Haw! Hee Haw!'*.

'Here comes my first choice as presidential candidate, His Excellency Doctor Professor Mister Mwansabamba Kabeji, President in Training of the People's United Republic of Peaceful Cabbages.'

'Why does he need a police escort?'

'To protect him from assassination!'

'Can a cabbage be assassinated?'

'Of course not!'

'Do the police know that?'

'Of course not!'

'Why not?'

'They're all cabbages!'

The cavalcade came to a halt, but the sirens continued to blare *'Hee Haw! Hee Haw! Hee Haw!'* But instead of a cabbage, out of the middle Mercedes stepped a big ugly beast. It stood there, blinking uncomprehendingly into the bright morning sun.

'Hee Haw! Hee Haw!'

'A donkey!' I exclaimed. 'Looks like Eunuch Kapimpinya!'

'Oh no!' moaned Velvet. 'The donkey has eaten the cabbage!'

13th September 2001

8.4 Dr Freddistein's Monster

IT was ghastly hot and humid in Cha Cha Cha Road, with storm clouds gathering overhead. To escape the heat, I took a short cut down a shady alley, round the back of the old Ambassador Funeral Parlour, now long deceased.

Or so I thought. For halfway down the alley I came to a sign saying *Kafupi Freddistein, Funeral Director.*

Curiosity opened the front door for me, so I stepped inside.

'Ah, Spectator Kalaki!' said a little fellow in a white suit, as he got up from his desk to shake my hand. 'I'm Freddistein. I've been expecting you.'

'Just a bit of rigor mortis in the joints,' I said. 'I could linger on for years.'

'Don't waste money on the pills,' he laughed, 'you'll have nothing left for the funeral.'

'So comfortable,' I said, as I lowered myself into a silk lined coffin and closed my eyes. 'Outside there are people fighting like rats over the smallest morsel, but in here its so peaceful. The government has really brought peace to Zambia.'

'And prosperity,' said Freddistein. 'Funerals are now very big business. With people dying at the rate of 300,000 a year, its created employment for thousands.

'Just imagine, ten years of coffins, all put in a line, would be 6,000 kilometres long! The line would stretch all the way from here to the World Bank in Washington.'

'Then they would really be able to see our progress,' I laughed, as I lay back comfortably in my coffin. 'But can this government really be re-elected after sending so many to the grave?'

'To heaven! That's why we were declared a Christian country!' chortled Freddistein. 'The government has saved all these people from earthly torment, and given them heavenly peace!'

'But if all the satisfied voters have gone to heaven!' I said, sitting up straight in my coffin and wagging my finger, 'only dissatisfied voters remain!'

'You're right!' he admitted. 'So I'll let you into the secret. The *Movement for Mobilising the Departed* is going to get the vote out from the graveyard. Three million dead voters! It's an inbuilt majority! The secret of re-election is resurrection!'

'I thought your job was to put them in the grave, not take them out!'

'Come with me,' he said, taking my hand to help me out of my coffin, and leading me into the mortuary. He pointed to all the smiling corpses resting happily in their coffins. 'You have now departed from Zambia, and entered Zombia, where election success depends mostly on timing. We shall be holding the election during Halloween, when all the zombies rise up from the grave. All we need is a leader for the *Movement for Mobilising the Departed.*'

'How about you?'

'Good gracious no!' laughed Freddistein. 'Only a zombie can lead other zombies!'

'So how will you find him?'

'Not *find* him! *Make* him! Not many people realise that I have a *Monster Making Doctorate* from the University of Blantyre,' he declared as he flung open the lid of a huge coffin. There lay a monstrous ungainly corpse, with swollen belly and limbs stitched clumsily together. Two rusty metal electrodes were attached to each side of its head.

'You really think this thing can become a great leader?'

'Only if he is truly representative of all zombies. So I have stitched together parts from zombies of every tribe, from different graveyards all over Zambia.'

'But is this leader a truly indigenous Zambian Zombie?'

'I have taken parts only from those bodies which were buried in Zambia more than two hundred years ago, before any foreigner arrived.'

'Two hundred years! Did you find a brain still in good condition?'

'That's been a problem,' sighed Freddistein, 'the brain is too tasty, and the worms go for it first. For the moment, I've had to substitute with cauliflower.'

'And what are the two electrodes for?'

'They are connected to a huge lightening conductor high on the roof. When the first storm comes, a massive spark of electricity will surge down into the body and then...'

As he spoke there was a huge crash and flash of light. Both Freddistein and myself were thrown backwards as the monster's coffin was blown apart. Then, as we watched, the monster slowly sat up with a creaky rasping sound, and opened its eyes.

'Er er, um um ah,' it said, with a terrible moan.

Freddiestein put his arm around the monster. 'There there,' he said kindly, 'you're amongst friends. You are going to be our great leader.'

'Owa glate reader,' said the monster slowly, trying to mimic its master. 'Er, um, so I yam notty a cabbagy.'

'Of course not,' said Fleddistein, 'you're a cauliflower.'

'Aaaghh,' cried the monster, as tears poured down its stitched and battered face, 'ah yused tuh have a glate blain.'

'Don't worry about that,' snapped Freddistein, 'you can use mine!'

1st November 2001

8.5 The Bus

'WHERE'S Evans this morning?' I asked Jimmy the newspaper seller, 'I need somebody to look after my galimoto.'

'Evans? He's gone for lunch in the bus.'

'Bus? What bus?'

'All the street kids round here live in the old bus behind the Post Office. Come with me,' he said, taking me by the hand, 'and I'll show you how the other half lives.'

As we rounded the corner we met the sorry sight of the rusting hulk of the old derelict bus, without engine, wheels or windows. On its side remained the peeling letters of the bus company, *Murderous Motorway Destinations*. On the backside was written *Trust in God, not the driver.*

'Last remains of the once proud MMD,' laughed Jimmy.

As we climbed up the skeleton steps, we came to the amazing sight of all the street kids, enjoying their leisure. Some played draughts and chess, while others were fixated on a game of bridge. Everybody was too engrossed to notice us.

I found Evans huddled in a corner, chewing on a baguette, and reading a copy of Rousseau's *Emile*. 'Can you make any sense of it?' I asked.

'Only just,' he laughed. 'It's a very poor translation. The meaning is very clear in the original French.'

'I suppose you missed out on school.'

'Yes,' said Evans. 'I've been very lucky. Without school or parents, I've been left free to educate myself.'

As we were talking, an untidy shambling old man climbed up onto the bus, stood at the top of the steps, and began shouting at the empty car park. 'Tiyeni! Tiyeni! Kwelani! MMD bus to Manda Hill!'

'Who or what is he?' I laughed.

'You shouldn't laugh,' said Evans, rotating his finger at the side of his head,' he lost his brains years ago. He thinks he's the driver of the bus! He's known as Kabeji.'

The slovenly monster seemed to hear his name mentioned, because he now turned slowly towards us, and began to growl at us in a low monotone ...

'Eee, eee, eeer, erum, erum, eee...'

'Is he trying to speak?' I whispered to Evans.

'He's making engine noises,' laughed Evans. 'He thinks he's starting up the bus, to drive to Manda Hill!'

'Eeeh, erum erum! I'm the new driver!' shouted Kabeji, sitting on an old bucket, and steering the bus with an imaginary steering wheel.

'Where's the previous driver?' shouted Jimmy, joining in the fun.

'Er, erum, erwa, Wabufi had to go to New York,' spluttered Kabeji, as saliva dribbled onto his battered unshaven chin. 'He's gone to to to to, to say thankyou to all the shuh shuh shuh shareholders, and vesters, and eh donors who have vested so much in this uhbus cuh cuh cuhmpany.'

'The bus has got no wheels,' laughed Evans.

'Er, ere, erum, erumrum,' replied Kabeji, revving up his engine, 'That's coz Wabufi was such a kind and generous man.'

'Generosity with other people's property,' sniggered Jimmy. 'Isn't there a special word for that?'

'Yes,' laughed Evans. 'Its called theft.'

'Shush,' said Jimmy, looking around anxiously, 'you can be arrested for saying things like that! Uzamangiwa bakaku-mvela!'

'So without any wheels,' Jimmy hooted, 'how are you going to get this bus to Manda Hill?'

Old Kabeji now tried to look stern and stood up straight. He drew in his fat belly, which caused his great baggy trousers to slip down. As he grabbed them back, his shirt flopped out of his trousers, and his wonky spectacles fell off his nose. 'What er, what um, what you don't realise,' he spluttered, 'is that ahrum, I am a leally a velly well organised disciplinarian...'

'Or a disorganised planetarium,' murmered Evans.

'And I shall use my dis dis discipline in training, I mean my training in discipline, to to to make sure that no more wheels are stolen...'

'There's none left to steal,' cackled Evans.

'... the Glate Wabufi has laid the foundation for our journey by giving us this chassis. He has made a start, and now we must look for some wheels to... erum, erum erum... there's lots of old lorries and spare wheels at Namboard...'

'It's a shame,' I said to Jimmy. 'What happened to him?'

'He used to be a real driver once,' said Jimmy. 'But he lost his marbles in a bad accident.'

'Namboard is the answer to all our plob plob ploblems, I am velly clear about that.., velly clear... erum, erum, er, er ...' he growled, as his eyes closed and he began to snore. Then he staggered and fell backwards off the bus. Jimmy moved quickly to the front to make an announcement.

'The trip to Manda Hill has been postponed until next March,' he laughed, as all the bus cheered. 'The driver has gone to look for some wheels.'

15th November 2001

8.6 Nomination Day

THE Supreme Judge sat at his Supreme Desk in the lobby of the Supreme Court, like a latter day Buddha.

Suddenly cries were heard outside, 'Kanono for ever!' Into the lobby strode King Kanono himself, followed by his Chief Bootlicker, Velvet Mango.

'I told you to have him here by 9 o'clock screamed little Kanono, stamping his high heels on the marble floor. 'We shall look like fools if he doesn't appear!'

'Sorry Your Excellency,' whimpered Velvet, grovelling on the floor, and trying to lick the king's boots, 'I thought you'd sent the helicopter.'

'Helicopter! We can't use that!' hissed the King, stealing a sidelong glance at the Buddha, 'I've told the old fool that this election is on a level playing field.'

Just then there were more cheers and ululations from outside, and the King and his Bumbling Bootlicker hastened back to the entrance to see what was happening. 'Candidate Kabeji!' roared the crowd, as a hundred party cadres carried an old bus chassis to the front of the Supreme Court.

'Isn't it marvellous to see the party machinery in good working order?' purred Velvet into his master's ear.

'Who took the wheels?' asked Kanono.

'Don't worry about that,' said Velvet, we've still got the party cadres.'

'Who took the engine?'

'We're better off without Western technology.'

On an old rusty bucket at the front of the bus sat the driver, an untidy old shamble of a man in a dirty brown suit. He pulled at an imaginary handbrake, opened an imaginary door, stepped out onto an imaginary step, and fell face down on the pavement.

The King frowned and dug his stiletto heel into Velvet's foot. 'Is this our Kabeji, or have you brought the wrong one?'

'Hooray!' cried the enthusiastic rented crowd, as the drums rumbled. 'Our Candidate! Our Kabeji! He has dropped from Heaven! Mphasao ya kwa Mulungu! Appointed by Kanono!'

As a thousand chitenges danced to the drums, so a thousand cabbages danced in the breeze. 'Who needs to capture hearts and minds?' murmured Velvet, 'when we can capture so many bottoms!'

The old brown Kabeji was helped to his feet, and began to climb the steps. 'My God!' whispered Kanono, as the monster approached, 'this can't be our Kabeji. Looks more like old Chakomboka!'

'He's dead.'

'So's this one,' retorted the King.

'A cabbage in the hand,' sniggered Velvet, 'is worth two in the vegetable garden.' So saying, he grabbed the confused old man by the back of the neck, and hauled him into the lobby, and in front of the Buddha.

'Name?' demanded the Supreme Judge.

'Er, erum, argh, aha, araghargh,' replied the old man, coughing and spluttering, as sticky globules of green gelatinous phlegm splattered onto the Supreme Desk.

'I'll put you down as a don't know,' said the Judge, moving his chair backwards to get out of range.

'His name is Loony Kabeji,' snapped Kanono. 'Just write it down, before I have you investigated for plotting a coup.'

'Yes Your Excellency,' shivered the Buddha, as his wobbly fat began to solidify like candlewax. He turned towards Kabeji, 'Hold this book in the air, Sir, and repeat after me...

'I being of sound mind...'
'I, being of Garden Compound...'
'do solemnly swear...'
'do seldom swear...'
'that I was born a Zambian citizen...'
'that I was born in Southern Michigan,'
'and my parents were born in Zambia...'
'and my parents were born in Gambia...'
'and that I am not too old...'
'and I shall do as I'm told...'
'to always say no no to corruption...'
'to follow Kanono's instructions.'

'Almost correct!' laughed the Buddha. 'I'm sure you'll get it right with a bit more practice. Now you can go outside and celebrate with your supporters.'

As they came outside the crowd cheered, and the shambling old monster raised one arm in the air and shouted *'This day's my last!'* So saying, he fell down in a heap.

'Your Candidate has announced,' Velvet shouted to the crowd, 'that *the die is cast!*' Then, turning to the party cadres he growled 'Get this corpse out of here!'

As the crowd began changing their tee-shirts and chitenges, in preparation for the next candidate, Kanono was busy climbing onto the cushions in his Mercedes. Suddenly he heard a gruff galumping sound right behind him. There stood the drooping flesh and slobbering mouth of the real Loony Kabeji.

'Where were you, you gormless old fart?' screamed Kanono. 'We had to do it without you!'

'Sol sol solly I'm late,' he spluttered, as saliva dribbled down his scarred and battered chin. 'I went to the Civ Civ Civic Centre by misteck.'

'Your not up to Kanono's standard,' jeered Velvet. 'You'll never be able to drib drib dribble like him!'

29th November 2001

8.7 Election Race

AS I joined the crowd outside the High Court waiting for the start of the Election Race, I found myself standing next to a man in a pinstripe suit, bowler hat and umbrella. 'Good gracious,' I said, 'you look like a British member of parliament.'

'So I am,' he laughed, shaking my hand and doffing his hat, 'Sir Meddlesome Meddlecraft of the Liberal Degenerates, and member for Lower Genitalia.'

'Spectator Kalaki, Senior Political Correspondent of *The Post*,' I replied, as I shook his hand. 'What brings you here?'

'I've been sent by the British government, to make sure your next Head of State is properly elected. Explain to me what is happening here.'

'What you see here,' I said, 'is the beginning of the Race to Plot One.'

'Horse racing? Like Royal Ascot?'

'No, its more like the London to Brighton race for vintage motor cars. Each party puts forward its own vehicle, and they race all the way to Plot One.'

'Just up the road! It'll all be over in five minutes!'

'No. They have to travel all round the country, and then back to Plot One! Winner takes all!'

'Good gracious! Are the roads good enough!'

'Oh yes. The government mends them once every five years, just for the Election Race.'

'Good gracious,' he said. 'I must put that in my report.'

As we were talking, the party cadres began to push their motley array of strange vehicles towards the starting line-up. 'Look at that one!' laughed Meddlecraft, pointing to a large tin trunk, 'no wheels at all!'

'The tin trunk is the symbol for the MMD, the Movement for Money Delivery,' I explained. 'It was made famous by the huge delivery of funds from the National Assembly to the Party Conference.'

'Is it still full of money?'

'Now it contains their presidential candidate, the famous Splutter Kabeji.'

'With the lid closed?'

'That's their election strategy. He's more respected if he's not seen or heard.'

'How are these vehicles supposed to move?'

'The supporters have to carry them. The more supporters, the faster you go! That's how you win the race!'

'But how do you get more supporters? Persuasive oratory? Promises? Charm? Humour? Manifesto?'

'Money!' I laughed. 'You have to buy them!'

'That's not allowed under British rules,' exclaimed Meddlecraft. 'The Foreign Secretary will take a very serious view of this. What other parties are in the race?'

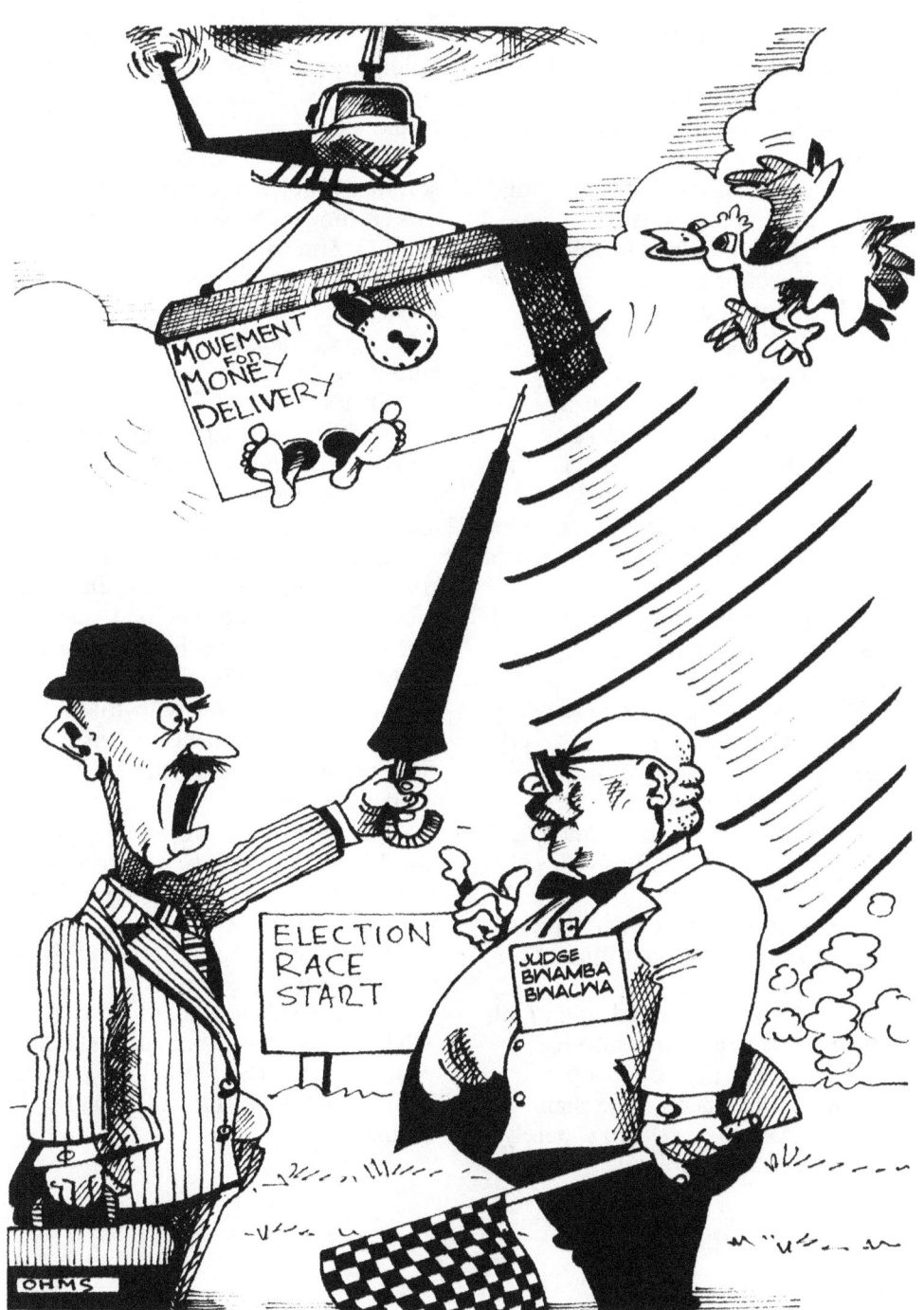

'That one down there is the Jumping Castle of the Up and Down Party. Its full of hot air.'

'What about the big wooden elephant?'

'That's the Forum for Deceiving Donors. It has thousands of supporters, but they're all pulling in different directions.'

'What about the big long boat with the dancing queen?'

'That's the Nalikwanda of the Agenda for Zero. It can't go anywhere, except on the flood plain.'

'Then the dancing queen can't go anywhere. Is this a fair race?'

'If we have early floods, the others could drown, and she would come in first!'

'And who's that going round and round the roundabout on a bicycle, waving a sword?'

'That's the notorious Cycle Mata, leader of the Panga Party. He's very experienced at destroying the supporters of other parties.'

'You can't have a level playing field with such skullduggery!' exclaimed Meddlecraft.

'And who are those two standing on that wooden cross and quarrelling with each other?'

'They have both called upon God to support their parties. But God, having been equally called upon by both parties, has decided to stand aside, and therefore to allow purely political factors to prevail.'

'The British government can't be giving money to church parties. It's entirely against the rules. And who's in the steel cage?'

'That's the leader of the United National Intolerance Party. They've locked him up to stop him running back to Zimbabwe.'

'Intolerance Party. This is intolerable! And who's that woman wearing a Scandinavian wig, and sitting in a sauna?'

'That's poor old Crone Kasote of the SDP, the Supporters Disappearing Party. She's known as the Swedish Candidate, because all her supporters are in Sweden.'

As we were talking Judge Bwamba Bwalwa raised his flag, and they were off! The race had started! Then there was a deafening whirring sound, and over the High Court swooped a helicopter with lowered rope. It scooped up the tin trunk, and flew off with it, as all the MMD supporters cheered.

Meddlecraft ran over to Judge Bwalwa and screamed at him. 'Did you see that! Call off the race! Is this what you call a level playing field? I shall put this in my report! Is this the way to elect a Head of State?'

Judge Bwalwa looked down at Meddlecraft with a bemused stare. 'In your country,' he said calmly, 'What is your procedure for electing the Queen?'

6th December 2001

8.8 A New Leaf

Sunday 23 December

I'm having such a nice time, *Dear Diary*, since my husband was adopted as a Presidential Candidate. Its lovely seeing him on TV, and all the posters saying *Vote Kabeji Mwalwemwalwe*.

I don't think I ever told you, *Dear Diary*, how it all started. It was a couple of months ago, I happened to bump into little Wabufi in London, when we were both shopping for high heels.

'How's poor old Kabeji?' he asked. 'Still in a mess?'

That was when I had the idea of getting my share from his Slush Fund, for Kabeji's medical expenses. 'I have to do everything for him,' I replied. 'Tell him what to do. Dress him in the morning. Do up his shoe laces. Change his nappy. The doctors say he may never recover. Dreadful, when you remember the man he used to be.'

Wabufi was so touched that he wrote out the dollar cheque on the spot.

The next morning I was still in bed at the Dorchester when the phone rang. It was Wabufi. 'I've been thinking about Kabeji,' he said. 'We need a Presidential Candidate!'

Monday 24 December

Dear Diary, I am so looking forward to Election Day, and becoming the First Lady! Just imagine, shopping in Rome and Paris for the latest Versace, and then flying on to Hamburg in the Presidential jet, and ordering the latest Merc for my dear darling husband.

But oops, *Dear Diary*, I nearly forgot to report the big event of the day! My visit to the starving handicapped orphans in Garden Compound! What a stench! Absolutely ghastly and stinking! I quickly threw them five million in a brown paper bag, and rushed back home to have a nice soak in my Jacuzzi. But my gold silk brocade suit is absolutely ruined!

Tuesday 25 December

Christmas Day, and I got the headline in *The Post*! **Fifty Orphans Injured in Scramble for Cash!** Marvellous! I phoned ZTV immediately, to cover my visit to the orphans in hospital. Unfortunately the chocolates made the children sick, because they'd never eaten such things before. They never will again, unless they survive to the next election!

Wednesday 26 December

Went to a mass rally of twenty-five people in Mutendere! It was marvellous! I spoke for five minutes, sensitising the masses to understand that hunger is a bad thing, and they should avoid it like I did. Then my darling Kabeji stood up and spluttered incoherently for another five minutes. How the crowd cheered! *'Alesosa Mwalwemwalwe!'* they shouted.

There's no doubt they want change. They don't want another clever man for president.

Then Wabufi spoke for half an hour. How eloquent! 'I have come here today' he said, 'to tell you that your government cares, and is aware that most of you are severely handicapped! Many are economically handicapped! Others are educationally handicapped! Or physically handicapped! As well as mentally handicapped!

'So vote for a handicapped man, one like you, who can represent your interests and understand your plight! This is what democracy is all about! Now is the hour! Never before have the handicapped been represented in Parliament, let alone in State House! Democratic principles demand that you be properly represented! This is your chance! Vote for Kabeji!'

Thursday 27 December

Its all over. My darling Kabeji has won by a landslide, over three million votes. Which just goes to show how very popular he is, because there are only two million voters. The Western observers can't even believe it, but Booby Bwalwa says that's because they can't understand African arithmetic.

Friday 28 December

Dear Diary, this was the day I'd been waiting for, being shown round State House by Wabufi. 'Aren't you supposed to be packing?' I asked him, 'we're planning to move in tomorrow.'

'As President of the Party,' replied Wabufi calmly, 'I shall be remaining here. The NEC has decided to put you temporarily in the servant's quarters, pending a decision on your duties.'

'There's something you should also know,' said my husband, bending down to look little Wabufi in the eye. 'I just pretended to be a cabbage, to trick you into adopting me. With immediate effect you are under arrest for misappropriation of state resources.'

'What!' spluttered Wabufi. 'Your stut stut stutter has dis dis disappeared! You have cheat cheat cheated me! I've been tricked! You are notty a cabbagy! I'll fix you! I'll break you! I'll break you for breakfast! For breakfast!'

'Breakfast! breakfast! Wake up! Wake up!' Sara was shouting and shaking my shoulders. *'Election Day! Get up!'*

'I had a strange dream!' I replied. 'So real!'

'Election Day! Who are you voting for?'

'The cabbage.'

'The cabbage!' she laughed, 'you must be joking!'

'The cabbage,' I replied, 'is going to turn over a new leaf.'

27th December 2001

8.9 Employment Opportunity
Advertisement in The Daily Sellout 24th July 2003

New Ministerial Opportunities

Introduction

Some recent ministerial appointments have recently been subjected to mischievous criticism from some infamous political failures and treacherous malcontents. These enemies of the state have made scurrilous claims that these appointments have contradicted national interests, or election commitments, or democratic principles, or even constitutional requirements.

In the interests of transparency, therefore, the government has contracted the services of the renowned human resources expert, Spectator Kalaki, who has been asked to explain the present fair and transparent system for the recruitment of ministers and deputy ministers.

The intention of this advertisement, therefore, is to make it clear that we have a democratic system of equality of opportunity, where all citizens are free to compete for selection into these positions of wealth and privilege.

New Ministerial Positions Available

Taking advantage of the latest budget overrun, the government is looking for applicants to fill sixty new posts for ten cabinet ministers and fifty deputy ministers.

Preference will be given to members of opposition parties, since members of the ruling party are already in government, or are otherwise incompetent, dishonest, or in jail.

Party Membership

A successful candidate from an opposition party will be required to immediately leave his party, renounce all the political ideals that he previously stood for, denounce his previous leader as morally bankrupt, and join the ruling party.

Personal Qualities

The successful candidate should be morally steadfast and upright, staunch in his political ideals, and loyal to his leader.

Educational Qualifications

An applicant should be highly educated, either with old Standard 4, or the modern equivalent of an UNZA degree.

An applicant who is able to read and write will be eligible for consideration for the higher post of cabinet minister.

Previous Political Experience

A minister normally has to be elected to Parliament. (However, in exceptional cases, where the applicant is completely inexperienced, or unelectable, or despised by the people, he may be nominated to Parliament.)

Applicants are therefore expected to have previous experience of how to buy votes in a buy-election, using such techniques as distributing blankets, tee-shirts, beer and bags of mealie-meal. Equally important are tactics of using ghost voters and multiple voting, ferrying of voters and stuffing of ballot boxes.

The applicant should also have experience of intimidatory techniques, such as the use of pangas for confiscating voters cards, or the use of police for tear-gassing enemies of the government.

The applicant is also expected to be well versed in strategies of using government personnel, vehicles, equipment and propaganda to thwart opponents who may try to use the buy-election to disseminate ideas which have not been officially approved by the ruling party.

Expertise in using machines to issue NRCs would be an added advantage.

Understanding of Ruling Party Policy

The applicant must be fully committed to the ruling party's fight against corruption.

Terms and Conditions of Service

The remuneration of a cabinet minister includes:

- *A salary of K80 million a year*
- *A rent free mansion*
- *Free house servants, gardeners and driver*
- *A personal-to-holder Benz with free mileage*
- *Cell phone with unlimited talk time*
- *Overseas education allowances*
- *Sitting allowance for sitting and doing nothing*
- *Per diem of $250 for shopping trips abroad*

The duties of a cabinet minister are to attend cocktail parties, and to explain to civil servants why the government has no money to pay their housing allowances.

A deputy minister's remuneration is different in that he is given a smaller house and smaller car. He has no duties at all, but is allowed to follow ZNBC cameras wherever they may go.

Gender Equality

Women are encouraged to apply, since government is keen to increase the number of women who are friendly with ministers, and who support male supremacy. Women who favour change are instead encouraged to seek employment with Women for Change.

How to Apply

Put this advertisement under your telephone at the side of your bed, and wait for the phone to ring at 3 o'clock in the morning.

Chapter 9
Religiously Irreligious

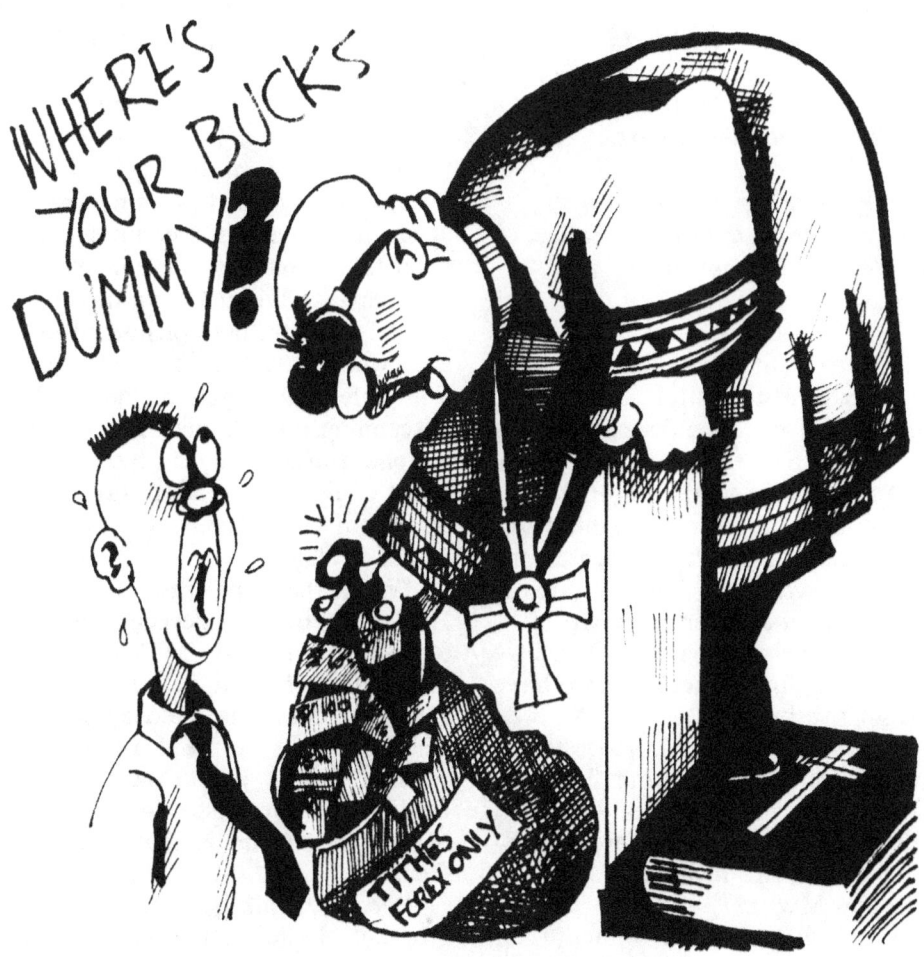

9.1 St Ignominious

IT was rather late when Sara and I slipped into the Sunday morning service at St Ignominious. The congregation was just beginning the Lord's Prayer ...

Christian Nation, which art in Zambia,
Hallowed be thy name;
Thy terror come
To us in Lusaka, as it is in Jerusalem.
Save us each day from daily dread,
And forgive our legislators,
As we forgive those
Who legislate against us;
Protect us from the Secret Police,
And deliver us from evil.
Amen

By now Father Mupulumpunshi was already in the pulpit, ready to begin one of his meandering sermons ...

'As we sit here this morning in the Church of the Most Magnificent Deity, many of you have been asking yourselves whether things have really changed for the better since we became a Christian Nation. Do we have Good Governance? Do we have God's Governance?

'Look into your soul, and ask yourself honestly. Was your faith shaken when you turned on your radio this morning, and heard that armed police had invaded the house of Bululu Mwila?

'Admit a small sinful thought! Didn't you say to yourself that it reminded you of the Mad Munshumfwa's Dictatorship, rather than the Good Governance of God?

'But I say to you,' he cried, raising his arms to Heaven, 'where is your faith? Where is your loyalty? Who are we, as mere mortals, to question the Most Magnificient Deity?

'I know what you thought!' he trumpeted, 'when the Chief of Police could not explain it, and the Minister of Home Affairs knew nothing about it!

'I can see it in your eyes,' he said, leaning forward and pointing an accusing finger at the congregation. 'You think that they are evil men, and that they are lying! Oh ye of little faith! Have you not considered that they were struck dumb by the sight of a miracle! The angels of the Lord descending on a sinner! The Great Shepherd descending on his flock! What could mere mortals say about an Act of God! Theirs was the silence of the lambs!

'When the Lord sends his Heavenly Police to descend directly to deal with sinners, he does not inform the Chief of Police or the Minister! Let alone the Magistrate! The Lord does not need a search warrant! I refer you to the Word of God! I ask you, where is the Magistrate's Court in the Book of Genesis?

'Do you think because the Heavenly Police found nothing, then the raid was a waste of time? Think again! If the Lord visits you tomorrow night and finds nothing, are you innocent? Instead of faith, he finds nothing! Instead of belief, he finds nothing! Instead of blind loyalty, he finds nothing! Then you are guilty! How then will you get to Heaven? Will you not go to Hell?

'So it was with Bululu Mwila. The Heavenly Police searched his house all night and found nothing. Neither bible nor hymn book. Neither prayer book nor liturgy. Neither rosary nor crucifix. Not even a picture of Our Lord! The house of a fallen sinner!

'Our Lord is a fisherman, and every night he must go on his fishing expeditions. But before you scorn a fallen sinner, ask yourself if you are ready to be visited by the Heavenly Fishermen.'

He raised up his eyes, and addressed the stained glass windows with fervour. 'But for the righteous amongst us, the Lord is our shepherd, and we are his sheep. We must follow him, and obey his every word. If we have blind loyalty and faith, then we need not fear the Heavenly Police.

'So that is my message to you today. Now all rise to sing Psalm 23.'

As the organ struck the first note, we all burst into song ...

The Lord's my shepherd, I'll not scream,
He makes me down to lie;
On Nondo's swing he tortures me
As guards wait close by

My house he doth invade again
And me to walk doth make;
Under the threat of pointed gun
Even for my Leader's sake.

Yea, when I walk in death's dark vale
Then I shall fear much ill;
For he is with me, and his rod
And staff are meant to kill.

Torment and terror all my life
Shall surely follow me;
And in Red Brick forevermore
My dwelling place shall be.

Dark clouds scurried across the sky as Sara and I hurried away from the church.

'What do you think to the priest's question?' I asked. 'Do you think God has really taken over?'

'Difficult to say,' she said. 'Either God or the Devil.'

10th August 2000

9.2 An Extraordinary Death

'YOUR old friend is dead and gone,' laughed Sara. 'I wonder if you'll be able to carry on without him.'

'You're right,' I said. 'He was the central character. I'll write one last piece about his funeral, and then just wait for my own.'

We were sitting on a gravestone at Leopards Hill, watching the coffin of Velvet Mango being lowered into its final resting-place.

'Do you know the story of what really happened?' asked Sara.

'I was told he got hit by a cabbage falling out of the presidential helicopter.'

'Hah!' laughed Sara. 'What would a cabbage be doing in the presidential helicopter?'

'Good point,' I admitted.

'According to the story I heard,' said Sara, 'Maureen was busy cleaning all the filth, rats and cockroaches out of State House, when she opened a cupboard and out fell his corpse.'

'Lots of skeletons in the cupboards,' I said.

'Probably more than this graveyard,' laughed Sara.

'Whose skeleton is this?' I asked, looking at the headstone where we were sitting. On it was written *Holdwell Shula, 1950-99.* Underneath was a memorial verse,

Wherever you be
let wind go free,
For holding a fart
Was the death of me.

'Very good!' I laughed. 'May his arsehole rest in peace! Maybe Velvet had a similar death, after being told to keep this mouth shut. With all his lies and hot air bottled up inside him, maybe he died of internal poisoning.'

'I thought he looked quite healthy, lying in his coffin,' said Sara.

'Hah! That's a good one! The guy's dead!'

'Looked better than you,' persisted Sara. 'Still a very smooth Mango. Not a wrinkled old prune like you. You're the one that looks more like a corpse!'

By now the mourners were lining up to throw earth onto the coffin, as the choir started up with a mournful dirge, and the priest solemnly intoned 'Ashes to ashes, dirt to dirt, filth to filth.'

Around the grave sat twenty-five women in black, wailing and shrieking and throwing themselves about, each being held down by a posse of relatives. 'Quite surprising,' I said. 'They all seem genuinely upset.'

'Understandably,' said Sara. 'Each thought she was the only one, and now each has found there are twenty-four others.'

Now we came to the moment we had all been waiting for, when the notorious Wabufi Kadoli climbed onto an anthill to deliver the eulogy.

'Former ministers, former ambassadors, former generals, reformed dealers, and former ladies and gentleman,' began Wabufi, 'It is

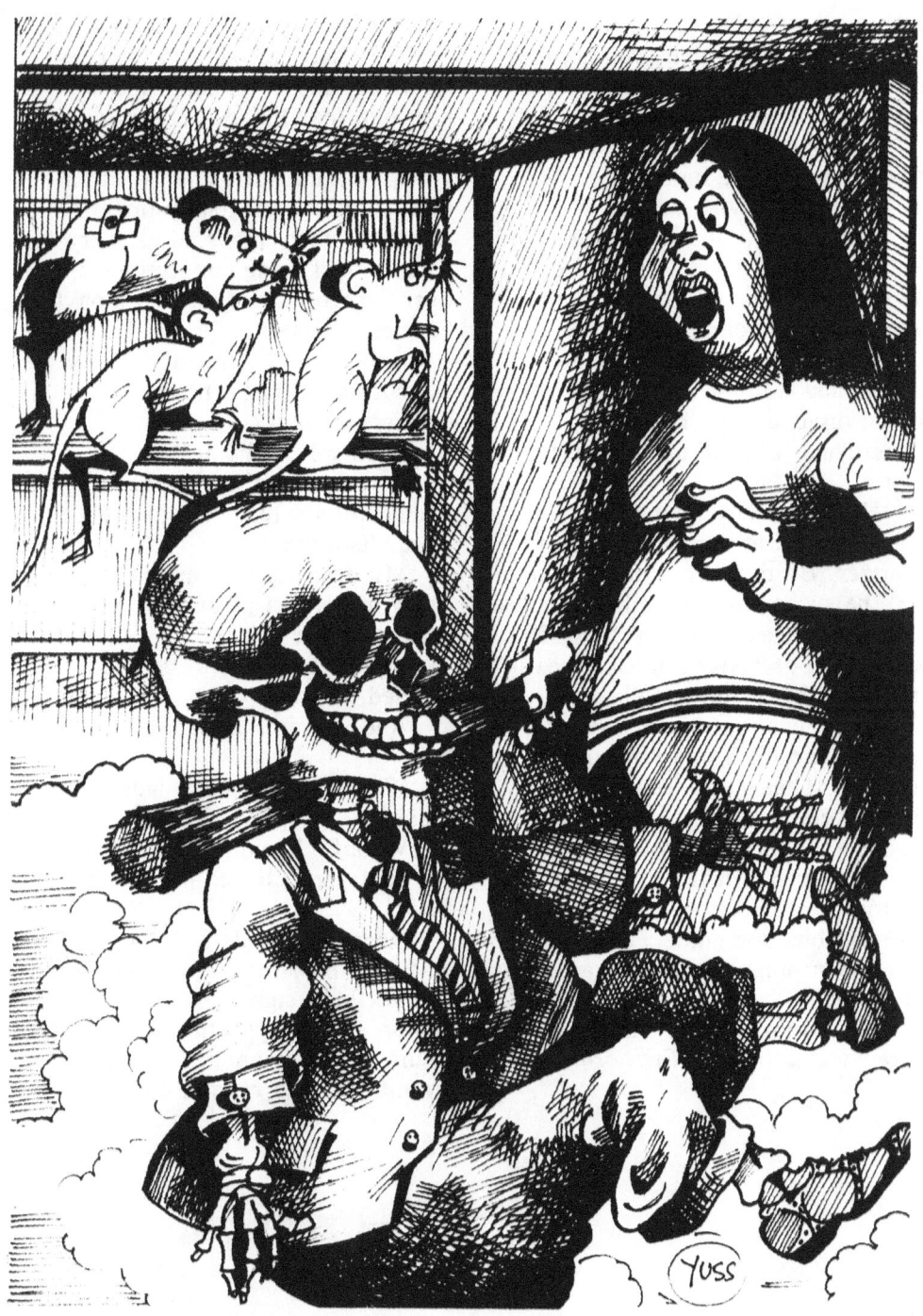

our sad duty today to say goodbye to our dear brother Velvet Mango, the most distinguished and talented liar this country has ever known.'

'Coming from Wabufi,' said Sara, 'that's high praise indeed.'

'I know many of us here are familiar with the illustrious career of Velvet Mango, but not many are aware of his humble origins. Velvet was born in Choma in 1944 of parents who were hardworking, honest and truthful. But despite this initial disadvantage, he was determined to make his way in the world.

'His first really momentous lie was achieved at the tender age of fourteen. By dressing himself as a girl, he successfully enrolled at Njase Girls Secondary school. As we all know, one of Velvet's most endearing traits was his inability to keep a secret. So every now and again he would share his secret with one of the girls. That's how Velvet was, often overcome by an overwhelming desire to unburden himself. And the girls felt so privileged to share his guilty secret. Because of these indiscretions, the entire Form Five were soon pregnant, as well as three of the nuns.'

'His autobiography,' chuckled Sara, 'was called *An Extraordinary Lie.*'

'The government,' continued Wabufi, 'soon recognised his talent for lying, and at an early age he was sent into the Diplomatic Service as an ambassador. It was there that his young and thrusting energy had a seminal effect, especially upon the wives of other ambassadors. Very soon he had made connections all over the world, and was promoted to Foreign Minister.

'And the rest is history. Today we are burying a man who is irreplaceable.'

When we got home, we saw a figure sitting on the veranda.

'Aarrghh!' I screamed, clutching at Sara, 'Its Velvet!'

'My dear Kalaki!' laughed Velvet, rising to his feet, 'You look as if you've seen a ghost!'

'You're supposed to be dead!' I shouted.

'And also irreplaceable,' added Sara.

'Who told you that?' laughed Velvet.

'Wabufi,' I said.

'And you believed him!' laughed Velvet.

'How did you do it?' I asked.

'I found that the death certificate had not been signed by a qualified doctor, so I'm appealing to the High Court. In the meantime, I've obtained an injunction to resume duties.'

14th March 2002

9.3 Prayer for the Departed

THE funeral service had already begun as I slipped into the back of Kabwata Preposterous Church, where the congregation was already in full song:

What a fiend we had in Deacon,
All his sins we had to bear,
What a privilege to bury,
For the bastard didn't care,
O what peace we had to forfeit,
O what needless pain to bear,
All his sins we had to carry,
For the bastard didn't care.

I spotted Young Sam at the back of the church, and went to stand next to him. 'They really raised the roof with that one!' I said. 'Its completely blown away!'

'Huh!' snorted Sam. 'The roof was stolen by the Deacon, when he was building his house in Badlands Extension.'

'The Deacon? Who's he?'

'He's the one we're burying today! How can you come to a funeral without knowing who's being buried?'

'Please be seated,' said the priest, 'as I call upon one of the church elders, Mr Malumbe Malumbo, to deliver the eulogy.'

'Dear Preposterous Brothers and Sisters,' began Malumbo, 'our Deacon came among us in 1991. We did not know his name, for he had so many names. But he praised the Lord in such chisungu chisuma, that we soon made him our Most Marvellous Deacon, and he became known to all of us as MMD.

'O my dear congregation, it wasn't long before he announced that he had received his instructions directly from God, so that he had no further need for the Council of Church Elders. The first divine instruction involved removing the stained glass windows, in order to give us better ventilation. Then he removed the church roof, saying that this would enable him to communicate with God directly, and enable our prayers to be heard.

'After that, he declared the introduction of fees for the Preposterous Church School, saying that it would help people to appreciate the value of schooling. Worst of all, he announced the Preposterous Housing Initiative, selling the priest's house to himself for ten gluders, and renting it to an official from the World Bank.

'We finally realised that we had allowed a Most Malevolent Devil into our midst. But our faith did not desert us, for we knew that the Lord would save us one day, and righteousness would finally prevail. So this morning let us bend our heads in the Prayer for the Departed...

Our Deacon, who art in coffin,
Cursed be thy name.
Thy end has come,
Because of evil done
In this church very often,
We shall never forgive the lackeys
You employed to trespass against us
And lead us into damnation,
For you are the devil
Who returns now to your kingdom
Of hell fire and torment,
For ever and ever,
Amen.

'And now,' said the priest, 'we come to the body viewing. Do not show your emotions inside the church, but please wait until you get outside. Do not be surprised or shocked at the appearance of the remains of MMD. For the Lord said that if thy right arm offends thee, then strike it off. In the case of MMD, most parts were struck off at an earlier stage, so that very little has remained for the administration of the last rites.'

As the congregation filed past the huge mukwa coffin, the choir continued with the earlier hymn...

We had our trials and tribulations,
We had trouble everywhere,
We were so angry and so desperate,
But the bastard didn't care.
So his friends they did forsake him,
Left him with his spoils to share,
With his friend in hell the Devil,
He will find no solace there

When we got outside, I said to Sam 'He looked so small in that huge empty coffin! I wouldn't have recognised him, except for the spectacles. And the whole head seems to have turned green.'

'It was eaten in the mortuary by the rats,' said Sam. 'So the undertaker decided to replace it with a cabbage.'

At the graveyard the coffin was brought to the graveside, the lid opened, and the corpse unceremoniously tipped into the grave. Then the coffin was put back in the hearse, which drove off.

'Good God,' I said to Sam, 'the coffin's gone back!'

'Yes,' said Sam. 'It belongs to a World Bank project. If we save on coffins we can export wood to Japan, and pay off our national debt by the year 5001.'

'And look at all that concrete!' I exclaimed, as a gang of men got busy with shovels.

'When you bury the devil,' laughed Sam, 'you need protection against resurrection!'

11th October 2001

9.4 Resurrection

SAM and I were sitting in the Strangers Gallery of the Great Cathedral at Manda Hill. We were about to witness the consecration of the new priest to preside over all their ancient and medieval rituals.

'Why is the priest in charge called the Speaker?' I whispered to Sam. 'Shouldn't he be a cardinal, or at least an archbishop?'

'This is a different sort of church,' explained Sam, 'Instead of priests, bishops and pope, here we have clerks, ministers and speakers.'

'But do they worship God or the Budget?'

'Here God is Money, and Money is God,' chuckled Sam. 'So they worship Money, which is the visible sign of God on Earth.'

'But that doesn't explain the Chief Priest being called the Speaker!'

'Money talks,' laughed Sam. 'The old God of the Israelites has not muttered a word for two thousand years. That's why the Pope keeps on quoting from old scriptures. But the God of Money is chattering all the time, through his representative on Earth, the Speaker. When the Speaker speaks, even the bishops tremble.'

Just then a shabby little figure shuffled in and crouched in front of the Speaker's Chair. 'Good God!' I exclaimed, 'is this odious little creature the new Speaker?'

'Of course not,' laughed Sam. 'This is Kwindi Chiwelewele, the church rat. He's been here so long, he was made the Chief Clerk. His job is to officiate over the proceedings, and then creep back into his hole.'

'Please be upstanding,' said Chiwelewele, to sing the Money Anthem...'

Stand and sing of Money,
market free,
Land of bribes and joy in unity,
Victors in the struggle
for the right,
We hold money tight,
Praise our Great Dollar,
Praise be, praise be,
Fat men we stand,
In the desert of our land,
For our Great Dollar,
Praise to thee,
Strong and free.

'There are two candidates for the position of Speaker,' continued Chiwelewele. 'Firstly there is Bumfutu Bapunda, who is well known as a silly ass. Standing against him is the most famous and distinguished son of this House, Mr Alesosa Mwelwamwelwa. Those who want Mwelwamwelwa should walk past the right side of my chair, for righteousness is next to godliness. Those who are misguided should walk on the wrong side.'

'What's that?' I asked Sam, pointing to the large copper cross hanging high on the wall.

'Copper crosses were used as money in pre-colonial days. That's the old Copper God.'

'And the tatty old cabbage, hanging on the cross?'

'Its popularly known as the Great Cabbage,' laughed Sam, 'but actually it's a big bundle of greenbacks. The new Dollar God.'

'It looks a bit tatty round the edges.'

'Chiwelewele is known to have a nibble, now and again.'

'And the motto underneath?'

'Continuity with change,' said Sam.

As we were talking, the members were filing back from voting. 'Look!' I said. 'Some have cabbage leaves sticking out of their pockets.'

'Dollar notes,' laughed Sam. 'They're already finding out how to get nearer to God.'

'Our new Speaker,' announced Chiwelewele, 'is the Right Honourable Alesosa Mwelwamwelwa!'

'Hear hear,' cheered the members, as they counted their dollar notes, and Chiwelewele dressed the new Speaker in skirt, cloak and long white wig.

'He has to wear the wig,' whispered Sam, 'to cover the panga scars acquired during his years as a party cadre in the Movement for Murdering Dissidents.'

'My first duty,' said the Speaker, 'is to lead the House in the Oath of Allegiance. 'Please bend the knee, and repeat after me...'

Our Dollar, which art in pocket
Hallowed be thy name;
Our tin trunks have come,
A new deal is done,
With Pajeros, to take us all to Heaven.
Give us each day our daily bribe,
As well as our government houses,
And imprison those who speak out against us,
For ours is the dollar,
the power and the glory,
With girlfriends
for ever and ever,
In bed.

'And now,' the Speaker solemnly announced, as he gave the sign of the cross, 'I do adjourn this House *sine die*, while I await further instructions from God the Kwacha, God the Dollar, and God the Holy Cabbage.'

What freedom it was to walk out from the fetid flattulent air of the Cathedral of the Holy Cabbage, into the fresh breeze outside.

'There's something familiar about the appearance of that new Speaker,' I said to Sam. 'He looks remarkably like the previous old villain. Same corrupted and rotting flesh!'

'You're right!' said Sam. 'They've had him resurrected! It's a miracle!'

'A miracle of God or Money?'

'In a Christian Nation,' laughed Sam, 'there's no difference.'

7th February 2002

9.5 Free Willy

'THE first lesson this morning,' said the priest, 'is from the Gospel according to St Kalaki, Chapter 1, verses 2 to 34.

'And in those days there lived in the land of Zambia a young man who was much respected, even by his elders. For he had a great brain that could comprehend all of the scriptures. And a great heart that could encompass the love of God. But most of all he had a great willy which was always willing to go anywhere. Which is why he became known as Willingo.

'And in those far off times, before the advent of political parties, there were limited opportunities for becoming prosperous without doing any work. So Willingo, like many a young man before him, decided to join the Church.

'And because of his great brain, thousands flocked to his church to hear his sermons. For he had developed great talents for justifying the unjustifiable, and forgiving the unforgivable, which are sure signs of a great philosophical mind.

'And because he took so many nuns as his wives, he was given the title of Archwilly, meaning that he stood high above all the other willies in the land.

'And because of his great heart, he used the enormous wealth from his collection plate to set up hospitals for the sick, and orphanages for his many children.

'But all was not well in the Church at that time, for in those days Zambia was a colony, under the domination of the Roman Church. All the old dried up foreign Pharisees from Rome were too jealousy of Big Willy, saying *Who is this young upstart who has taken all our nuns, leaving us to sleep alone?* And so they began to poke their long thin critical noses into his affairs, because they didn't have any affairs of their own.

'So one day the Pharisees summoned Archbishop Willingo before them, accusing him of taking wives outside the Church, although he had taken solemn vows to provide his services only to the Brides of Jesus, since he was married to the Church.

'But the Archwilly answered them calmly, saying that *Barren women come to me and I make them fertile, for it is written that every pregnancy is a gift from God.*

'Then the Pharisees, having their own Scripture quoted to them, cursed and tore their hair at the insolence of this young priest, saying *You are also accused of witchcraft. We have reports that your willy has been flying around like a nyanga, exercising free willy instead of following God's will, and entertaining whole convents in a single night. We are sending you to be disciplined by the Holy Godfather at the Vendetta in Rome.*

'And so the Archwillingo travelled

all the way to the enormous Castle of the Vendetta, and joined the three thousand other people waiting to see the Holy Godfather. Some had been waiting for thirty years, for the Godfather, like the Church itself, was now old, bent, deaf, incoherent and immobile. Critics claimed that he had died years ago, but priests still came and kissed his ring, claiming to see signs of life.

'But God had favoured Willingo, for it came to pass that after only twenty-five years he was called before the Inquisition.

'And the Chief Inquisitor said unto Willingo *You are charged that you did travel to New York to marry two thousand brides of the United Fornication Church, which is not recognized by the Holy Roman Church. So the Holy Godfather has granted you a divorce.*

'And Willingo answered him, saying *How can he grant me a divorce when he doesn't recognize the marriage? And how can a divorce be necessary if we aren't married? And who can grant a divorce when neither husband nor wife have asked for it? And if the Holy Godfather grants a divorce when this is absolutely prohibited in the sacred doctrine of the Roman Church, will he not surely go to Hell?*

'And for this heresy Willingo was banished to the Australian Outback and chained to Ayer's Rock. But by the time he died, Free Willy had managed to fertilize a thousand kangaroos, thus founding the first congregation of our beloved Church of Sexual Liberation.

'We now bow our heads in prayer for Free Willy...'

Our Willy, who art in trousers,
hallowed be thy name,
all praise is Sung,
when she has come
and the Earth has moved like Heaven.
Give him each day his daily bed,
and enjoy all his ecstasies
as we enjoy all those
who press them against us.
And lead us not into redemption
but bring back our Willy
His power and his glory
for ever and ever.
Amen

15th August 2002

Chapter 10
Strange Encounters

DEMOCRACY RESTAURANT
TODAYS SPECIAL "STRANGE ENCOUNTERS MENU

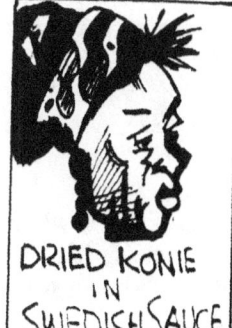
DRIED KONIE IN SWEDISH SAUCE

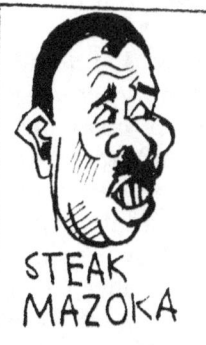
STEAK MAZOKA

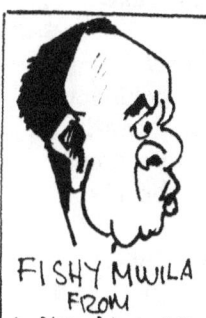
FISHY MWILA FROM LAKE MWERU

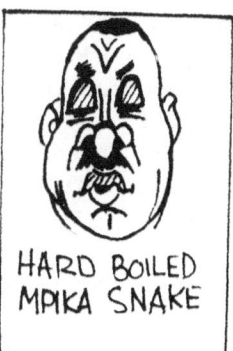
HARD BOILED MPIKA SNAKE

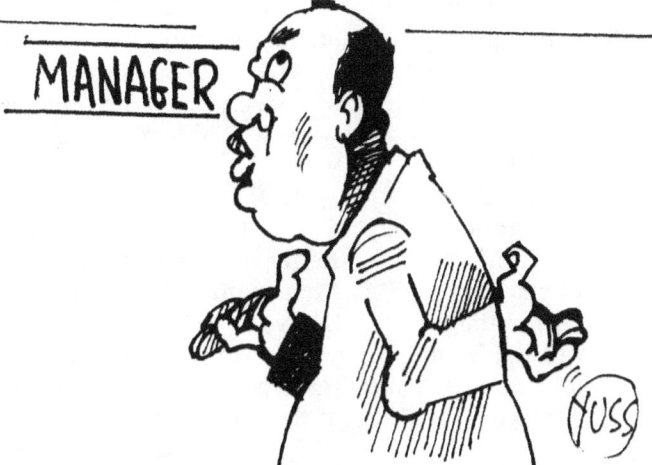
MANAGER

10.1 Mr Forgettable

YESTERDAY Sir Fred sent me to interview the new President of the United National Intolerance Party.

'Come in and sit down Kalaki, he said and ushered me into an armchair. Cigar? Whisky?'

'I've always been fascinated by your name,' I said, 'Frantic Coma? How did you get a name like that? From a missionary?'

'Not at all,' he chuckled. 'It's a nickname from when I worked at the Barley Bank. We used to make whisky out of barley.'

'But why Frantic Coma?'

'They used to say my behaviour was frantic in the morning, but in the afternoon I would fall into a coma.'

'Frantic until you got the first whisky?'

'Exactly,' he chuckled, taking a puff from his cigar and a gulp from his glass.

'So what was your original name?'

'No idea old chap. Long time ago. All that whisky affects the memory.'

'So how long did you last at the bank?'

'I'm not quite sure. One day I managed to sober up, and found I'd been fired some three years earlier.'

'Last week you even forgot which party you're the president of.'

'Ha, Kalaki, I knew you'd bring that up. It was a slip of the tongue caused by a mere slip of the brain. How could I forget that I'm President of the Movement for Milking Donors?'

'Not the United National Intolerance Party?'

'Ha ha, just joking Kalaki. Wanted to see if you could spot the mistake.'

'But you didn't go to Sesheke to support them?'

'Bit of a muddle on that one, I'm afraid. I accidentally went to Serenje, due to a typing error.'

Just then the phone rang, and Frantic answered. *'Who? Who's speaking? Benefit? Whose benefit? ... Oh, my wife, Benefit! Then why didn't you say so? ... No need to take that tone, I'm doing my best ... Anybody can forget a name ... Who didn't come home last night? Me? Are you sure? Never mind, dear, I'll come home tonight.'*

'That's the trouble, Kalaki, when you own so many houses. Difficult to remember which one is home. Now what were we talking about?'

'Your bad memory.'

'Oh yes, now I remember. Have another brandy.'

'We're drinking whiskey.'

'Much the same thing. Where were we? Where am I? Who are you?'

'Kalaki from the Post.'

'Quite right. Make sure you don't forget it, I thought you were Old Munshumfwa for a moment. Do you know, he always used to sit where you're sitting now. He was sitting in that very chair when he saw the light at the end of the tunnel.'

'A great man. He never let the

facts interfere with his point of view.'

'Who?'

'Old Munshumfwa.'

'Quite right. Trouble with Munshumfwa was that nobody could tell him anything. Nobody dared to say he'd got his chair the wrong way round. He was always looking at where he'd come from, back down the tunnel. So the more he went up the tunnel, the smaller the light became.'

'So what about the present government? Has it gone further up the same tunnel?'

'No, it has managed to reverse all the way out. But now it has gone round and round the same roundabout until it has run out of petrol. Or was that Castro?'

'I wonder, with such a bad memory won't it be difficult to be President of the United National Intolerance Party?'

'Not at all. Old Munshumfwa went mad because he couldn't forget his disasters. I was elected leader to help them forget their past. They spent so long in the tunnel that some of them are still having nightmares.'

'So are you changing the name of the party?'

'Yes. It's now the United National Investment in Politics. I bought the party at the last Congress.'

'Is it possible to buy a party?'

'Under multi-party democracy, even parties have been privatised. Party members can be bought very cheaply, so it's quite easy to buy the whole party. It can make a very good investment.'

'Collecting the rent on Freehold House!'

'Not only that. There's always the danger that the old UNIP could come back, and re-nationalise private property. So I took over in order to protect my investments.'

Just then the phone rang again.

'Hullo, I'm Frantic, who are you? ... Fleddie? Fleddie who? ...Have we met? ... Merger? ... Monopoly of Mobocracy Dictatorship?... OK, I'm on my way.'

He turned to me as he staggered towards the door, holding up the empty bottle. 'I can see light at the end of the bottle. I'm off to get another one.'

'Another bottle?'

'No, another party.'

27th July 2000

10.2 Sir Frantic

I was sitting in my Kabulonga Penthouse when Spectator Kalaki came to interview me for *Hardtalk*, on the BBC.

'Sir Frantic Coma,' he began, 'to what do you attribute your great success in becoming the new President of Zambia?'

'Ah ha, Kalaki,' I chuckled. 'When I last met you, you were just an ordinary journalist on *The Post*. I should ask the secret of your success!'

'I'm the one doing the interviewing!' laughed Kalaki. 'Let's start from the beginning. Two years ago you took over the leadership of the United National Intoxication Party. How did you do it?'

'Money and brains,' I explained. 'That's the secret of my success. I bought the party for a few crates of beer and a hundred teeshirts. Quite a nice little investment!'

'But I'm told it was difficult at the beginning. You lost a series of by-elections. Said the wrong thing at public meetings. Held your nose when meeting the lower classes.'

'Ha ha, so you heard about that, did you? You see, I belong to the new upper class, who have never been able to tolerate ignorance or the stench of poverty. That's why I decided to change the whole system.'

'The democratic system?'

'Exactly. Previously Zambia had a system of one person one vote. Even ignorant people with no education had the same vote as a clever fellow like me. It was a system of counting heads, irrespective of content.'

'So you've changed all that?'

'Of course. Now Zambia Limited is just another company, and I am the President because I am the one with the brains and the capital. The ordinary workers just shut up and do as they're told. They're much happier that way, because they're not intellectually capable of decision making.'

'In the past they had the vote.'

'Exactly. Being foolish people they elected people equally foolish as themselves. Being poor and lower class, they elected people of the same sort. First we had an impoverished schoolteacher in charge. After that even worse, we had a bus conductor from a very small minibus.'

'So how did you change the system?'

'It was quite simple really, for a brilliant person like myself. I set up Zambia Ltd as a company on the London Stock Exchange, and sold shares at a thousand dollars per square kilometre.'

'So you were able to buy the voters in the 2001 elections?'

'Exactly. I bought the voters for 100 dollars each. Other parties were offering only a bottle of Mosi, so obviously I won with a landslide victory.'

'And you made clear that they would never have the vote again?'

'Oh yes. I have always been ruthlessly honest and straightforward when explaining my brilliant ideas. I told them that I am rich and clever, and they are poor and stupid, and therefore they should hand the country over to me.'

'So then you closed Parliament, transferred the Judiciary to the Police Force, and set up a Board of Directors to run the country! Didn't you have trouble with the IMF and the Paris Club?'

'Ha ha. They were the ones who got the poor little Bus Conductor into trouble. He was always begging from donors to repair his bus. And they were always making him consult the passengers on which direction the bus should take. Obviously he lost control of the bus.'

'Donor funding was all a mistake?'

'Of course. What we needed was investment by clever business people. But investors demand political stability. They don't want the uncertainty of pandering to the voters' whims, and government changing every five years. Already I've got investment pouring in from Slavery International.'

'So what is the system for government administration?'

'I just run the business side, from this Kabulonga Penthouse. I've brought back that man Evelyn Hone for supervising the police, putting down riots, and that sort of thing. I've installed him in State House, or Government House as we now call it.'

'I must congratulate you, Sir Frantic, on your recent knighthood...'

Back to the present: Spectator Kalaki has just arrived at Freedom House to interview the new President of UNIP. He is greeted by loud snores. Frantic Coma is fast asleep in his armchair. An empty whisky bottle lies by his side ...

'Wake up! Wake up!' shouts Spectator Kalaki. 'Time for the interview!'

Frantic wakes up with a start, and stares at Kalaki with bleary bloodshot eyes. 'Ah, Inspector Lakaki, there you are! I wash just shaying. I wash given my knighthood by the Queen, for shervices to the Blitish Empire!'

24th August 2000

10.3 Popular Choice

ON Tuesday the family went out to the Democracy Restaurant for a grand New Year's Day lunch. Of course the usual confusion broke out when the waiter brought the menu, which was almost as complicated as a presidential ballot paper.

'I'll have the Mazoka steak,' I said. 'Why don't we all do that, to keep it simple and get the food quick?'

'He's just trying to save on the bill,' sneered Namukolo.

'Typical of Dad,' said Kupela. 'Takes us to the Democracy Restaurant, and then starts bossing us around!'

'Mazoka steak is boring and unimaginative,' laughed Sara, 'and as tough as an old boot! Probably fell off the back of a railway wagon! I'm ordering the Dried Konie with Swedish sauce.'

'That's like old string,' scoffed Aunty Irene. 'I'm having the Miyanda Snail with Pompous Dressing.'

'Yaliwe and I will try the Fishy Mwila from Lake Mweru,' said Luwaya. 'I should avoid that,' said Towani, 'I've heard its very nasty and poisonous. I think I'll play it safe, and just pick a bit of cabbage from other people's plates.'

'What about the Tembo ostrich?' asked Yumba.

'I always find Tembo bland and tasteless,' advised Yaliwe. 'More suitable for invalids and diabetics.'

'Then I'll be adventurous,' laughed Yumba, 'and try the Hard Boiled Mpika snake.'

'If you can stomach that,' said Towani, 'you'll swallow anything!'

'So that's the order,' I said to the waiter. 'And while we're waiting, can you bring a couple of bottles of the house plonk?'

It was a good job I ordered the wine, because we waited endlessly for the food, until we had entirely run out of wine, and even run out of Mwanawasa jokes. We were getting rather irritable.

'This is worse than voting,' Luwaya complained, calling over the waiter. 'What's the delay?'

'Sorry sir,' said the waiter, scurrying towards the kitchen. 'Your food's coming just now!'

Sure enough, within a minute the waiter reappeared bearing a huge copper serving dish, which he placed in the centre of the table. Then with a great flourish he lifted the lid, revealing a huge boiled cabbage.

'Is that it?' shouted Luwaya.

'That's the food you ordered. Is anything wrong sir? You seem a bit upset!'

'Of course we're upset!' I shouted, standing up and catching him by the throat. Where's my bloody Anglo American steak? I didn't come here to eat rotten cabbage! Bring the manager immediately!'

Within a couple of minutes a shambling figure arrived, shifting around within his sloppy suit. An incongruous mixture of subservience and arrogance. 'I'm the manager, Booby Bwalwa,' he said, as his eyes surveyed the ceiling. 'What's your problem?'

'We ordered the food hours ago,' I shouted, 'including a Mazoka steak. But after waiting for hours, this waiter has brought nothing except a boiled cabbage.'

'I have been doing this job for the past eight years,' he said. 'Are you trying to tell me my job?'

'Tell you your job!' shouted Luwaya. 'We're only asking you to bring the food we ordered!'

'Couldn't organise a beer party in a brewery!' sniggered Namukolo.

'Couldn't organise a vote in a polling station!' laughed Kupela.

'So what's your explanation!' I demanded.

'You have to understand things from my point of view,' said Bwalwa, keeping his left eye on the window and his right eye on the door. This is the Democracy Restaurant, where we always respect majority opinion. That's what democracy means.'

'Never mind democracy,' shouted Aunty Irene. 'What happened to my slimy little Miyanda snail?'

'You were the only person to order snail,' explained Bwalwa. 'In addition to the one snail, this table also ordered one ostrich, one prawn, two fish and two steak. But three people clearly and specifically ordered cabbage, which was therefore the popular choice by a clear majority. Individuals must respect the decision of the majority. So there's your meal! The cabbage! Bon appetit!'

'Its all our own fault,' I said, turning to the others.

'We could all have had the steak, if you'd only listened to me!'

'Oh shut up!'

'Let's just try to make the best of it.'

So we swallowed our pride along with the cabbage, and another couple of bottles of plonk to try to wash away the nasty taste. By then everybody in the restaurant had made the same mistake, and the air was growing foul with the sickening stench of flattulence.

And as it turned out, we were lucky to get out of there. As we reached the car park, the whole place exploded in a ball of flame. Somebody must have lit a cigarette. As we drove home, explosions could be heard all over Lusaka.

'They're all celebrating the popular choice.'

'Yes,' said Yaliwe. 'We must brace ourselves for the Year of the Cabbage.'

3rd January 2002

10.4 Strange Encounter

I was busy looking for shoe polish at Melissa supermarket in Kabulonga, when I heard a chirpy little voice from the bottom shelf.

'Kafupi!' I laughed, 'I didn't expect to find you here! Aren't you afraid of being seen?'

'I'm too far below eye level,' he chuckled, 'nobody notices me!'

'Aren't you supposed to have ten bodyguards to protect you from the people's gratitude?'

'The bootlickers have all disappeared,' sighed Kafupi. 'That's why I'm in here, looking for some polish for my high heels.'

Just then a young woman greeted me as she walked past. 'You must be Charles Chabala! I recognized you immediately from the picture! I did so enjoy your piece in the *Post* yesterday, about the bacteria taking over! How clever! How witty! But you look so pale, compared to the photo!'

'Just a bit of harmless skin fungus, supplied free of charge from the City Market,' I said, as I shook hands. 'Let me introduce you to my friend, the famous Wabufi Kafupi,' I said, turning round to introduce him. But there was nobody there.

'Never mind,' she laughed, as she moved off with her trolley. 'I'm sure you'll find another friend.'

'Pssst!' came a voice from under the cabbage in my trolley. 'Quick! Let's get going!'

'I'll pay for the cabbage next week,' I shouted across to Mr Gallopolous, as I galloped out of the shop with the trolley.

'Don't worry,' he shouted back, 'its quite worthless.'

'That was a close one,' laughed Kafupi, as I wheeled the trolley back to his house. 'You could easily have been lynched if they'd realised you were really Kalaki, and not Chabala!'

'If I was the one in danger,' I laughed, 'why did you hide under the cabbage?'

Twenty minutes later we were having a cup of tea in his large empty sitting room. He looked like a little cockroach, sitting in the corner of his huge white leather armchair. He was busy trying to pick off the worms and parasites that had fallen from the cabbage, which were now threatening to eat him instead.

'What are you doing nowadays?' I asked.

'Bit of bible reading,' he said. 'Never found the time before. Always talking about it, but never actually did it. Always had a pastor handy to give me a quotation.'

'No writing?'

'Nothing. Can't afford the writers anymore.'

'Any regrets? D'you think you chose the right person to take over?'

'Oh yes! Marvellous! Morleen and I are both political engineers! We're working together marvellously. We consult on the phone on a daily basis.'

'Morleen? You mean she's the one in charge? Just like Cycle Mata said!'

'Exactly. I employed Cycle Mata to say so, so that nobody would ever believe it!'

'So what's the job of Mr Mwanamwanamwana Stustustutter?'

'Him, poor chap. I left him in charge of the MMD, the Matrix for Money Diversion.'

'So what's Morleen in charge of?'

'She's in charge of Morleen's Money Donations?'

'An NGO?'

'Exactly. It's only the NGOs that can run the country nowadays. Donors are only willing to give money to NGOs, because government has been taken over by the Matrix. They won't give money to corrupt ministers, who were elected in corrupt elections, which they corrupted themselves, in order to get their filthy snouts in the Zamtrough.'

'But Stustutstutter says he's going to get rid of collcollcolluption!'

'A corrupt system cannot cleanse itself!' laughed Kafupi. 'The whole thing has to be thrown out, like a rotten cabbage!' He picked another worm from his lapel, and flicked it onto the floor.

'So what's the alternative?'

'You're not listening. The alternative is Morleen. The Morleen Educational Initiative receives the donor funding for education, and distributes school books. Similarly the Morleen Health Initiative distributes medicines to hospitals. The Morleen Housing Initiative builds new houses. And so on. She acts instead of government, collecting the funding, and deciding how to spend it!'

'So if she's in charge, what is the job of Stustustutter?'

'He's now the First Lady, with a purely ceremonial function of cutting ribbons, opening party conferences, making meaningless speeches, and telling lies at corrupted by-elections. None of his antics will matter, because all power is vested in Morleen's Initiative.'

Just then there was a knock at the door and in came six policemen. 'Mr Wabufi Kafupi, you are under arrest for stealing a supermarket trolley. Since the trolley has four wheels, it is classified as a motor car, so you cannot be given bail.'

'What! It doesn't even have an engine!'

'You are also charged with stealing the engine!'

'Half a minute,' I interrupted. 'I'm the one who took the trolley!'

'You shut up,' said the police officer. 'You're not the one we want to arrest!'

Kafupi stood up, fastidiously flicking yet another worm off his jacket. 'This damn cabbage,' he said, 'has really brought bad luck.'

29th August 2002

10.5 Cherise

YESTERDAY afternoon I must have dozed off, after washing down a cheese sandwich with a couple of beers. But I was woken by a persistent knock on the front door. Damn, I thought to myself, dragging myself reluctantly up from the sofa, I wonder if its a sin to murder a Jehovah's Witness.

'Kalaki!' she screamed as I opened the door. 'Cherise!' I gasped, as she threw her arms around me in a rib-cracking hug. Then she pushed me away at arm's length, examining me more closely.

'My darling Kalaki! How I've missed you! 106 days away! I was saving myself for you! Those young boys didn't interest me, I need somebody more mature!' She pulled me towards her again, and gave me a little kiss on the end of my nose. 'My crinkled cackling Kalaki, I just love all of you!'

'Nonsense,' I laughed, 'you just love my sense of humour!'

'Your sense of humour and your lovely littul beard, they tickle me all over!'

'Come and sit on the sofa,' I said, taking her hand, 'and we'll have a bit of tickle!'

'Where's Sara?' she said, looking round.

'Don't worry,' I said. 'She's away at a women's meeting, discussing how to control husbands.'

'You've been a naughty boy,' she murmured, snuggling up close, slipping her hand inside my shirt, and her tongue inside my ear. 'You didn't come to meet me at the airport, or the lunch at State House.'

'I wanted you all to myself,' I said, as I toyed with her shoulder straps, 'and those people are such boring frauds.'

'Yes,' she giggled, 'They've already given me a diplomatic passport. What d'you think they're up to?'

'Probably trying to involve you in a bit of old-fashioned import-export. There was a time when our diplomatic bags used to attract sniffer dogs from all over the world. But tell me, what are you really going to do?'

'Actually,' she said, 'I want to use the Big Brother concept to improve television in Zambia.'

'What!' I said. 'The original idea was a sort of nightmare dreamed up by George Orwell in 1949, where TV cameras would peer at us everywhere. The Big Man could become Big Brother, using the camera to control everything! No escape from the watchful eye of totalitarian government! You could even be locked up for refusing to eat cabbage!'

'Hhmmm,' she murmured. 'That's what I like about you, Kalaki. Your brain remains intellectual, even while your other parts are getting romantic!'

'Be careful what you're playing with! It can become a top-down tool for control and subjugation.'

'It depends who's in control,' she

giggled, pushing my head down onto the cushions. 'A nice bit of bottom-up reverses the normal power structure.' She sat on top of me and looked down, saying 'Let's play it bottom-up. We could put cameras in the offices and bedrooms of our rulers! See if they really do as they promise! See who's licking boots at State House! See when they pass the brown envelopes! See how much an opposition MP actually costs!'

'That would be a real bit of accountability and transparency!'

'Yes,' she said, as she loosened another button on my shirt, 'take their clothes off, and see how fat they've been getting at our expense. While the ribs are showing on my poor dear Kalaki!'

'We could peer beneath their fat gluttonous bellies,' I laughed, 'and expose the parts that they themselves haven't seen for years! Isn't it strange that the priests are opposing Big Brother's potential for revealing sin?'

'They're in two minds. On the one hand they were so glued to the screen for three months that all the church services had to be officiated by church elders, but...'

'But on the other hand,' I suggested, 'they're worried that one day the camera will come to them, and peep inside their cassocks!'

'That's right,' she said slowly as she stroked me thoughtfully, 'Big Brother can just grow and grow.

'Aarrrggghh!' I screamed, pointing at the screen, 'that's us on TV!'

Panic! We were still re-arranging ourselves when in strode Sara. 'Ah ha,' she cried triumphantly, 'caught you at it! I've got the camera connected to my cell phone!'

'You've got it all wrong!' I gasped. 'This is Cherise...'

'That's not Cherise!' snorted Sara. 'That's Chileshe from No. 82, across the road.'

'Cherise is the English pronunciation,' said Chileshe, as she quickly glided out of the room...

I woke up with a start. 'Caught you sleeping on the job again!' Sara was shouting, 'you're supposed to be writing that project proposal!'

'Sara, my darling.' I said, rousing myself sleepily from the sofa. 'Thank God you're back! You've just rescued me from a very tricky situation!'

11th September 2003

10.6 Bloodsuckers

WE had all been sitting for an hour at the Ministry for Child Abuse when finally into the Conference Room waddled the Minister, the fat and fatuous Mr Andrew Mosquito, followed by a sinister bunch of lackeys in dark shades.

'Strange name,' I whispered to Sam. 'He's far too big and fat to be called Mosquito.'

'Perhaps the size of brain,' Sam suggested.

'Please sit down,' said the Minister, apparently not noticing that nobody had stood up. Then, as he lowered his huge posterior into the high throne at the head of table, a lackey stepped forward and plonked a brown paper envelope in front of him. The Minister quickly scooped it up, into his jacket pocket.

'What was that?' I hissed to Sam.

'Sitting allowance,' Sam chuckled. 'Every time he sits down he's given two hundred pins.'

'What about sitting on the toilet?'

'Then its two hundred pins plus two toilet rolls.'

'Does he really need two toilet rolls.'

'Its strictly a matter of protocol,' Sam explained patiently. 'One for a deputy minister, two for a minister, and three for a vice-president.'

'Three for a vice-president?'

'Because we get so much out of a vice-president.'

As we had been whispering, another lackey came and put a tray of bread and wine in front of the Right Honourable Mosquito. He immediately closed his eyes and put his hands together, saying 'As a Christian Nation, let us pray,

Oh Lord, protect my friends here
From the deadly sin of jealousy
As I swallow this bread and wine
On their behalf.'

So saying, he opened his eyes and swallowed the delicious croissant in one gulp. Then he lifted the glass of wine to his nose, which seemed to grow longer as the wine quickly disappeared.

'He sucked it up his nose!' I gasped. 'Was it wine or blood?'

'Depends whether its been blessed,' said Sam.

'I have called you all to this Press Conference this morning,' began the Mosquito, 'to announce that all schools are closed indefinitely, with immediate effect, as part of the War on Corruption. It has been found that parents have been corrupting headmasters to buy school places, and corrupting the examiners to buy exam papers. This is what caused the previous government to become infiltrated by little criminals who couldn't read or write.'

'But isn't education a human right?' asked an NGO representative, apparently bent on undermining the government.

'Firstly,' he said, angrily thumping

a tattered law book onto the table, 'we are a government of laws, and this Constitution does not give the right to education. Secondly, and perhaps more important, what was happening in our schools was never anything to do with education.'

'So how shall we develop?'

'Ah, the President went all the way to China to ask that very question.'

'And what did they tell him?'

'They told him,' Sam whispered in my ear, 'not to waste his meagre resources on expensive trips to China.'

'They told him,' said the Minister, 'to find new resources to exploit.' As he spoke, his nose grew longer, then suddenly lashed out like the tongue of a chameleon, clasping onto the neck of a notorious *Times* reporter, the despised Mr Craven Bias. The blood was drained out of him in a few seconds, reducing him to a dried raisin, which was then carted off by one of the sinister lackeys.

'Blood!' cackled the Minister, as his nose shrank back, and his belly swelled. 'This is our remaining resource. We have sucked out the copper! Sucked out the taxes! Sucked out the pension funds! Sucked out the housing allowances! Now we shall suck out the blood, and export it to America!'

'Even the Christians will oppose this,' whimpered the man from *The Mirror*. 'Isn't blood a human right?'

'Hah!' laughed the Minister, again thumping the battered book, 'Where does this Constitution give you the right to blood? Nowhere, my friend! I've been through the whole book very carefully, and the word blood is not mentioned even once!'

'So is this the new development policy we've been waiting for?' squealed the frightened little mouse from *The Mail*.

'Exactly,' said the Mosquito, licking his lips and looking around for another juicy neck. 'We of the Movement for Mosquito Development have actually been making good progress. In the last ten years we have multiplied the mosquito population from fifty million to a hundred billion. This is our other great resource, leading to the doubling of the death rate for under-fives, and huge savings in the Health sector. Now we can move to the final phase, of exporting blood!'

'But what about human rights?'

'Always thinking of yourselves!' exploded the Minister, 'instead of thinking of others! What about freedom of movement, and freedom of association for the poor little mosquito!'

'I think,' sniggered Sam, 'they've finally worked out a strategy for winning the next election!'

13th November 2003

10.7 Professor Supple

THE massive door of the Yunza Lodge opened slowly, revealing a young woman in jeans and bare feet. 'Spectator Kalaki?' she asked. 'The Vice-Chiseller has suggested that you join him on the veranda.'

A grey and stooped old gentleman peered over the top of his Wall Street Journal, then rose slowly from his breakfast table, and held out his hand. 'Spectator Kalaki, how nice to meet you at last. I'm Professor Rubble Supple! You seem surprised!'

'Er errum,' I said, 'I was expecting a younger man!'

'Don't worry, young Kalaki, my body may be rubble, but my mind is still supple! Please sit down! Have some Oxford marmalade and toast! Have a cup of French coffee! Have some delicious Mauritian oysters!'

'Good gracious,' I said. 'You live well!'

'I invest in myself,' he cackled, 'for a very high rate of return!'

'That's what I wanted to talk to you about,' I said. 'Your method for resuscitating an ailing university.'

'To save a university from turning to rubble, you have to be supple. That's how I got my name, Professor Rubble Supple.'

Just then the same buxom young woman came bouncing down the veranda towards us, carrying a message for the Great Professor. But as she knelt down respectfully at his side, her buttocks suddenly plopped out from the back of her over-stretched jeans. She stood up quickly, trying to squeeze them back in, as I stood up to help.

'You should have bought the next size,' I said.

The Professor sighed as we both watched her waddle back down the veranda. 'That really sums up what's wrong with this country...'

'What d'you mean?' I exclaimed. 'She's perfect! You'll never find anything more supple than that!'

'If you'll just let me finish,' snapped the Professor, 'I was referring to your suggestion that she should buy a bigger size. Where's she going to find the money? She's just a student of Communication Technology ...'

'You mean she carries messages...'

'... she's a student who I am employing at twenty pins a month. She'll probably have to work here for another thirty years to pay off her tuition fees.'

'So she'll never afford new jeans.'

'Precisely,' he said, slipping another oyster down his throat. 'Education is about adapting to your environment. That's the subtle meaning of being supple. She must accept her jeans as part of her given environment, and adjust her size accordingly.'

'Starve herself a bit.'

'Exactly.'

'I remember a time,' I said, 'when university students were educated to make the environment better, not just adapt to what they find.'

'You're out of date, Kalaki. That

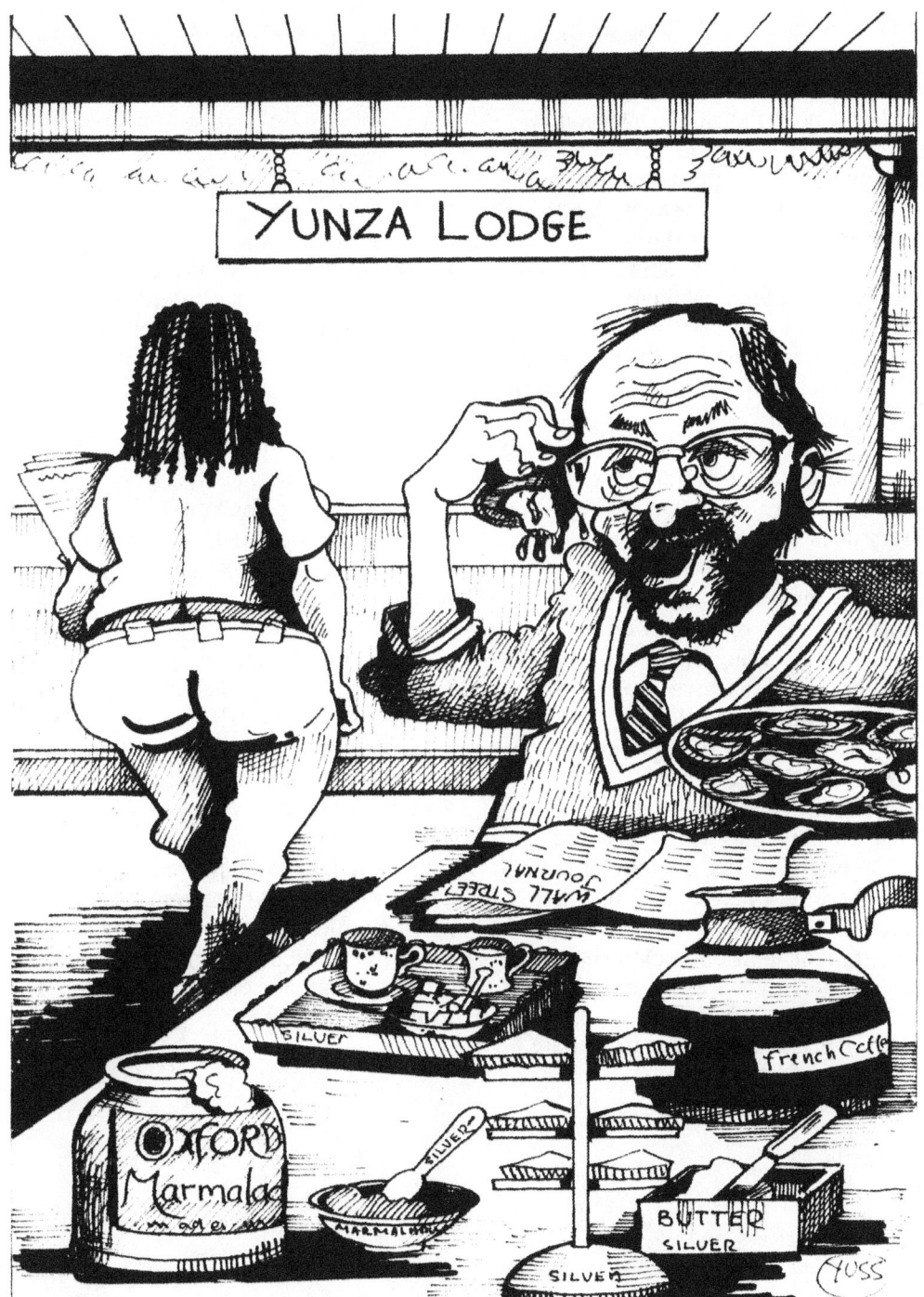

was back in the old days, when we used the university to create the new ruling class.'

'And now that job's been done?'

'Exactly. Now we just train these students to assist the new ruling class by carrying their messages, licking their boots, counting their money, rigging their elections, finding legal loopholes, defending them on treason charges, and that sort of thing. Nowadays we just train the lackeys.'

'So you don't train them to think for themselves?'

'My dear Kalaki,' he said, putting his hand on my shoulder, 'nothing could be more dangerous. The ruling class does the thinking. It is a fundamental principle that our students must not question decisions taken by duly authorised bodies.'

'But this ruling class will not live forever. How shall we produce the next generation of rulers?'

'The members of this new ruling class send their children to universities in England and America. That's where they learn how the world really works, so they can come back here and take over from their parents. This is very costly for the government, and obviously there's nothing left over for Yunza.'

'But these Yunza students still believe that a certificate from here will be a passport to the ruling class!'

'That's why we insist they pay their own fees. Government can't waste money on such a hopeless venture!'

'So you advise them to invest in themselves!'

'In a democratic country, its important that everybody feels they have an equal chance to succeed. And when they fail, they must blame themselves for making a wrong investment. We don't want them blaming the government.'

'What about yourself,' I asked, 'when you were at university, did the government pay for you?'

'Oh yes,' he laughed, 'I must have cost them a hundred thousand dollars!'

'And did they get a good return on their investment?'

'Of course,' he cackled. 'I've saved them millions!'

In the distance we began to hear the sound of gunfire and screams, and a bullet whistled overhead. 'We still have some rebellious students,' he said, 'but I have employed a duly authorised authority to make them more supple, so they are better able to adjust to their environment.'

'More supple, but more rubble,' I suggested.

6th November 2003

Chapter 11

Contempt of Court

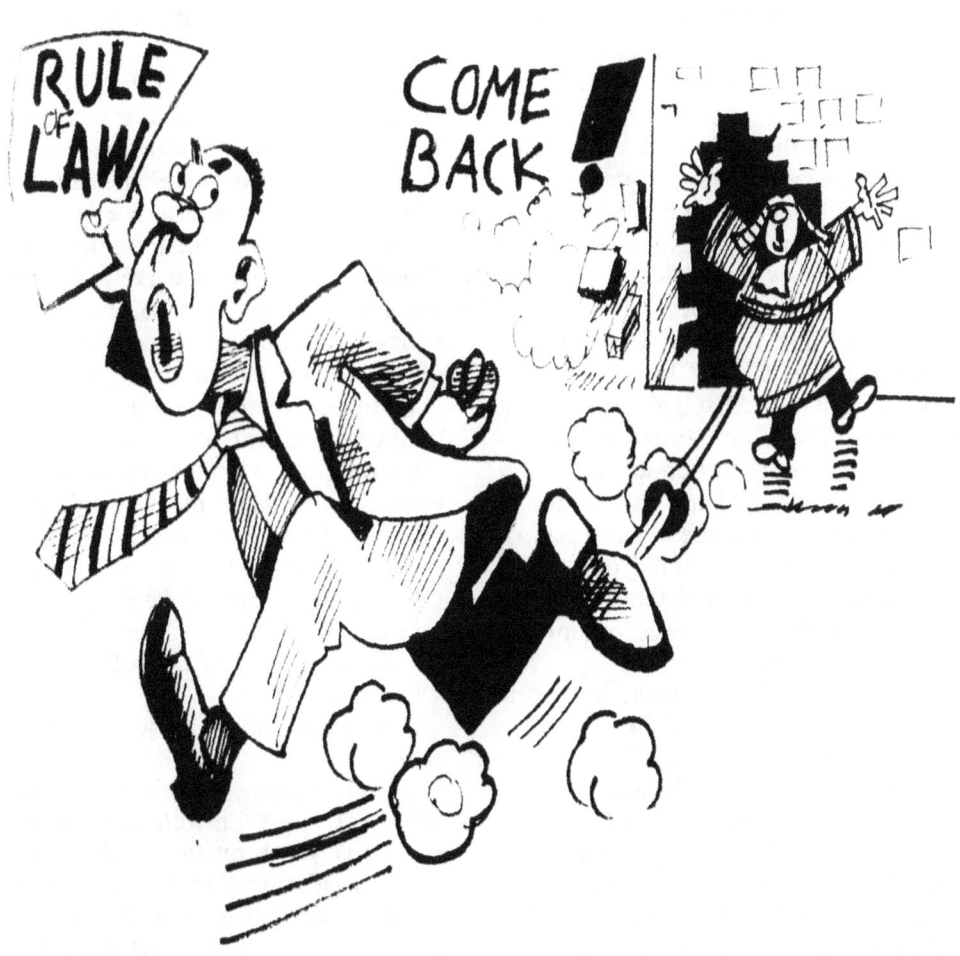

11.1 The Merry Judge

IT is Thursday morning at the High Court. Sam and I are sitting in the gallery, waiting for the first case to begin. 'What's on the menu this morning?' I asked Sam.

'Petitions!' he chuckled. 'They're always amusing!'

'And who's the Judge?'

'Justice Gregarious Merry. Loves a good joke! If something has to be laughed out of court, he's the one to do it!'

In came the Judge, as we all stood up and bowed. 'That's right,' said the Judge with mock solemnity, 'we must all show respect for the absurdity of reality, and try not to laugh. Ha ha! Where's the first case?'

'A petition from Mr Chipuba Chiwelewele, Chief Clerical Officer at the Ministry of Miseducation and Delinquency, Your Lordship. He is asking the court to uphold his administrative decision that Grade Seven pupils with the lowest exam marks should be admitted to secondary school, and those with the highest marks must leave school and seek employment.'

'Put him in the witness box so he can speak for himself!' laughed the Merry Judge. 'I am sure he has a most entertaining explanation!'

'Your Lordship,' began Chiwelewele, 'I am basing my position on the Education Policy, Article 104(c), which states that education must be provided according to the needs of the child. Obviously it is those who have done badly in the exam who need more education, whereas those who came out top are the ones better qualified to seek employment. Following your confirmation of the rightness of my decision, I also seek a court order compelling police to arrest the thousands of protesters who have been hurling bottles at Ministry Headquarters.'

'Ho ho ho,' laughed the Merry Judge. 'The most amusing petition I've heard all week! But the petition is denied because under the law the school selection criteria are determined by the Examinations Council, of which you are not even a member. You are a mere clerical officer with no say in the matter at all. However, I request the ACC to investigate whether you are a member of the Movement for Manpower Disposal, and whether any of your own children have recently failed Grade Seven. Next case!'

'I am Sub-Inspector Chipumbu Chiwelewele,' began the next petitioner.

'So many Chiwelewele!' I whispered.

'A whole family of idiots,' replied Sam.

'I am seeking a declaration from the court,' said Chiwelewele, 'that cars must drive on the right-hand side of the road, and that it is illegal to drive on the left. Cars drive on the right in most countries of the world, and under Interpol Agreement Clause

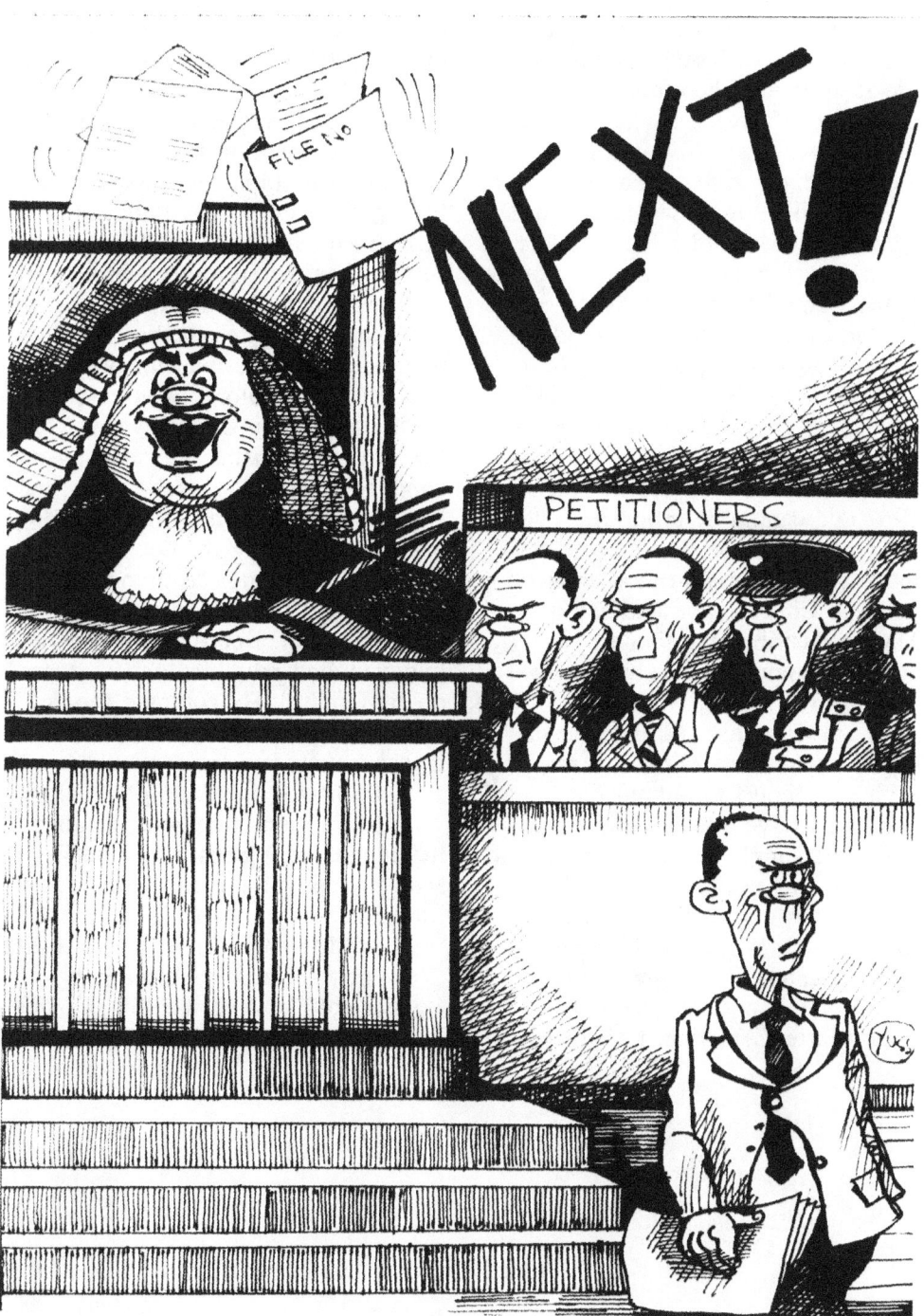

257(z) the government has agreed to the international harmonisation of traffic systems. Therefore I ask the court to confirm the legality of the fines amounting to five million gluders which were levied on motorists in Cairo Road last Saturday morning, and to order the arrest of all the motorists presently hurling bottles at the Central Police Station.'

'Green means stop!' cheered the court, 'and red means go!'

'I need hardly tell you,' chuckled the Judge, after we had all stopped laughing, 'that the rules of the road are laid down in the Traffic Act of 1967 and cannot be arbitrarily altered by a sub-inspector. Therefore I ask the ACC to investigate the connection between Chiwelewele and Moto Market Distributors, who are currently importing left-hand drive cars from America. Next case!'

'I am Chipunsha Chiwelewele, Chief Engineer of ZESCO. I am asking the court to uphold the decision I have already taken to lower the supply voltage from 230 to 110 volts, as used in America and most of the world. This is in conformity with World Trade Treaty of 2001 Chapter 23 Paragraph 491(q), which allows cheaper electrical imports from America. I also seek a court order for the arrest of all rioters presently besieging ZESCO Headquarters.'

'Nice try,' laughed the Merry Judge. 'The petition is denied because decisions on voltage are taken by the Energy Council, and are not the business of the Chief Engineer. The petition has therefore been brought to a wrong court. However, I request the ACC to investigate whether the petitioner is a salesman for Michigan Machine Distributors. Next case!'

'I am Chituku Chiwelewele, Chief Lunatic at Chainama Hospital. I have conducted research which shows that Lusaka residents drink more beer than water. I am asking the court to support my decision to pump Mosi beer through the pipes previously used for water. Beer is clean and hygienic, and produced under proper quality control. By contrast, Lusaka water is infested with bacteria and faecal matter, and is notoriously used as a means for distributing cholera.'

'The petition is denied,' laughed the Judge, wiping his eyes, 'but I send my congratulations to the Mosi Marketing Department. Next please!'

'I am Mwelwa Chiwelewele, Chief Clerk of the National Assembly.'

'Oh no!' laughed the Judge. 'This is going to be the best!'

31st January 2002

11.2 Where is it?

'MR Cycle Mata,' said the Judge, 'According to the evidence put forward by Inspector Waffle Watumpa, you secretly stole the Rule of Law from the government, and have been driving it around as if it were your own.

'But evidence from many witnesses has shown that you have never had anything to do with the Rule of Law. Whenever you wanted to fix your enemies, you always hired your own gang of thugs. I therefore absolve you of any charges of ever having had anything to do with the Rule of Law, and you are accordingly acquitted.'

'Thank you My Lord. I should just like to say how grateful I am for my stay in Kamwala Prison. Despite my considerable previous experience, I had never before managed to meet so many thieves and criminals in such a short time. I have recruited them all into my party, and we will soon be in a position to take over the government.'

'Splendid!' laughed the Judge. 'That's what we mean by democracy in this country!' But then the Judge turned more seriously to the Clerk of the Court. 'I am very concerned about how this case was botched by this baffled buffoon, Inspector Waffle Watumpa. Weren't the Police supposed to have brought the Rule of Law here, as an exhibit of the stolen property?'

'My Lord!' exclaimed the Clerk of Court in alarm, 'the Suspector General has always been very clear that the Police will never have anything to do with the Rule of Law!'

'Then why wasn't it brought by an officer of the court?'

'It would set a disastrous precedent, My Lord. The Rule of Law has never had any role in court proceedings!'

'Really? Why's that?'

'Due to the constitutional separation of powers, My Lord. We are concerned with administering the law, not with ruling. That's the job of the executive. Once a court concerns itself with the Rule of Law, it would set a dreadful precedent. All previous judgements would be wide open for appeal, because of evidence obtained under torture. Even those hanged would have to be dug up, resuscitated, resurrected and retried. Both the cost and the smell would be inestimable.'

'So where is the Rule of Law now?'

'It was Mr Bigwig Abashi who claimed that Cycle Mata stole the Rule of Law. So perhaps he's the owner!'

'Now we're getting somewhere!' exclaimed the judge. 'Call Bigwig Abashi!'

An ancient little bald fellow hobbled arthritically into the witness box. 'Are you the owner of the Rule of Law?' asked the Judge.

'I am the Very Right Honourable Sir Doctor Bigwig Abashi, constitutional lawyer with three degrees, and currently Minister of Perks for Supply.'

'Yes yes,' said the Judge irritably, 'we know all that. The question was whether you are the owner of the Rule of Law?'

'Ha ha,' cackled the wrinkled old lizard, 'I'd never fix my enemies if I bothered with that! The Rule of Law is supposed to be kept in a safe place, locked up in the cells of the Shushushu.'

'Has the Rule of Law committed an offence?'

'Its not that. But if the Rule of Law were set free, the Shushushu themselves would immediately become unconstitutional.'

'My God,' said the Judge. 'All cases would come to court! Bring the Supreme Shushushu here, to confirm that he really has the Rule of Law under control.'

'We can't do that, My Lord, the Shushushu does not officially exist.'

'I forgot that! Then how shall we know if the Rule of Law has escaped?'

'Already there is worrying news from Livingstone,' said Abashi gravely, 'where the former master race from Down South have established the New Krugersdorp, for those who want to relive the fantasies of the Rider and the Horse. But union leaders are refusing to allow their workers to be ridden and whipped, and the Sin Hotels are instead having to import their own horses. If the Rule of Law rears its ugly head there, we could lose our investment, and the racist monsters might all go home.'

'Even if Cycle Mata is not the culprit,' said the Judge gravely, 'it certainly looks as if the Rule of Law might have escaped. I must get to the bottom of this. Bring the Chief Government Spokesman.'

So now the fat face of Mr Bedstead Dimba blinked uncomprehendingly at the court. 'Mr Dimba,' said the Judge sternly. 'Can you tell us the whereabouts of the Rule of Law?'

'I can assure you,' said Dimba slowly, 'that the Rule of Law is safely in the custody of the government.'

'Yes,' snapped the Judge. 'But who governs the country?'

Dimba paused, scratched his head, and looked at the ceiling. 'This country is governed,' he said, 'by the Rule of Law.'

16th May 2002

11.3 The Trough

'SPECTATOR Kalaki,' grunted the Judge, 'you were supposed to appear before this court four weeks ago. Where have you been?'

'I was taken into psychiatric care, My Lord. But now I've been discharged.'

'Not by this court, you haven't!' laughed Justice Pig, squealing with delight at his own remark. 'Mr. Judas Musangu, you're the prosecuting counsel, remind me of the charge on which we intend to find this man guilty.'

'Defamation,' declared Musangu, as Judge Pig put his long snout into the trough at the front of the bench, pulled out a few dollar bills, rolled them around his mouth, and swallowed them with a loud belch.

'You mean *Defamation, My Lord*,' declared the judge sternly. 'We must have respect for the judiciary.'

'My profound apologies, My Lord,' said Musangu, bowing low towards the bench, and slipping a few dollar bills into the trough to show even further respect.

'That's more like it,' declared the Pig, leaning back in his chair and stroking the hairs on his belly with genuine affection.

'This man Kalaki,' continued Musangu, 'defamed my respected client, Mupupu Kafupi, the internationally famous thief. Kalaki misused his column in the gutter press to declare that the Thief is the President.'

'Not that the President is the Thief?'

'Same thing, My Learned Lord. If God is King, then King is God.'

'Your argument is based on a very sound constitutional principle,' agreed the Judge. 'So proceed with questioning Kalaki, then I'll sentence him.'

'Spectator Kalaki,' began Musangu, 'did you write in your column that the Thief is the President?'

'But why did Kafupi imagine that he was the thief to whom I referred?'

'Come off it, Kalaki. He is the most famous thief in the land. He rose from stealing tomatoes and school certificates, through to stealing a widow's inheritance, then government houses, until in the end he stole a whole copper mine. A capitalist dream of rags to riches. No den of thieves is complete without a picture of their Paramount Thief on the wall. When you mention the Thief, everybody knows you mean Kafupi.'

'That is what they infer, and not necessarily what I imply. But if people think I refer to Kafupi, how have I insulted him by calling him President?'

'Really, Spectator Kalaki, don't get smart with me! You know very well that in the last ten years all our hospitals and schools were destroyed, starvation stalks the land, and millions have died. A time of bogus trials, false imprisonment, torture, murders and assassinations. You know that if the person responsible for all this can be found, he will certainly be hung. And yet you have suggested that my client, the popular and famous Mupupu Kafupi, was actually the one responsible!'

'But did not little Kafupi prance around in high heels and flashy suits, calling himself President? Am I the one responsible for that?'

'Mr. Kalaki, really. You know very well that Kafupi was the President of MMD, the Matrix for Money Diversion, an association of common thieves and criminals. He always made it very clear, in word and deed, that he was President for only MMD, and not for all Zambia.'

'Perhaps so. But wasn't he actually elected as President of Zambia?'

'Really, Kalaki, try to be honest with yourself. You are the very one who has argued that the Constitution was hijacked, elections rigged and votes bought. You claimed that the whole of the electoral process was so corrupted that we did not have a President of Zambia, but only a President of Corruption! Now you dare to come here and claim he was duly elected!'

'But everybody else thought that little Kafupi was the President!'

'Half a minute,' interrupted Judge Pig, lazily lifting his drooling snout out of the dollar trough, 'I happened to hear what you were saying. I was the very judge who presided over the election petition. I can therefore tell you authoritatively that Kafupi was not the man who was elected as President. We never discovered quite who it was that was elected, only that it was not Kafupi.'

So saying, the Judge's snout fell back into the trough, and rummaged around, coming up with another mouthful of dollars. 'Look at this,' he grunted. 'This is the very evidence on which I based my earlier decision.'

At this point Musangu emptied the contents of a large brown paper bag into the trough. 'And in view of this further evidence,' continued the Judge, 'I find Spectator Kalaki guilty of defamation, and sentence him to be locked up. Locked up! Locked up!...'

Wake up! Wake up!' I opened my eyes, to find Sara sitting at my bedside in Chainama. 'You've been discharged! You weren't insane, after all! Ngulube was on the take, just as you said!'

'I know,' I replied. 'I saw his snout in the trough.'

11th July 2002

11.4 The Cookie Monster

'YOU have been brought before this court, Spectator Kalaki,' said Judge Nyangalala, 'because you wrote in *The Post* of Thursday 1st August 2002 that the President is a Cookie Monster. How do you puleeed?'

'I plead with you, M'Lord, not to buy the newspaper if it upsets you so terribly.'

'I'm getting fed up with the lack of respect for this court,' snapped the Judge. 'I could cite you for contempt!'

'I do share your concern, M'Lord, with the increasing number of people who are becoming contemptuous of your court, and indeed of the whole judiciary.'

'You'd better cut the cackle, Kalaki. You are here to explain why you claimed that the President is the Cookie Monster, when you knew very well that the Cookie Monster is nothing more than the figment of the imagination of an American TV producer. As a professional journalist, your job is to report facts, not fiction.'

'That is your opinion rather than fact. But I shall nonetheless report what you have said, since I don't agree with your opinion.'

'Don't get smart with me!' screeched the Judge. 'I just want to know whether you can prove, as a fact, that the President is actually the Cookie Monster.'

'It is a fact that I was told so by Kermit the Frog.'

'What!' scoffed the Judge. 'Is not Kermit equally a figment of Jim Hansen's imagination? As a professional journalist, did you not try to verify this information from an independent source?'

'Oh Yes, My Lord. A State House source confirmed that our beloved President can't keep his hand out of the cookie jar, and everybody calls him the Cookie Monster.'

The Judge put his head wearily into his hands. 'Mr Sleazy Surmiser, you're supposed to be the Prosecuting Counsel. Please continue the questioning. This Kalaki is giving me a headache.'

'I put it to you, Kalaki,' said Surmiser, rising to his feet, 'that you knew very well that Kermit was just a slimy little green frog, a compulsive liar trusted by nobody. Obviously he was not a reliable source of information.'

'I must protest, M'Lord, at this line of questioning. What the Prosecuting Counsel obviously doesn't realize, and not many people know, is that this same Kermit was our President for ten years. People voted for the Frog as the only way of getting rid of the Mad Munshumfwa. Kermit was a very accomplished TV performer, and nobody at that time realised he was just an American puppet, with long fingers and an empty head.'

'But you knew! So what's your point?'

'The point is that I had to respect his information that he had put another puppet in his place. It takes one puppet to know another!'

'Hah!' said Surmiser, smacking his lips. 'It now seems, M'Lud, that this case is assuming a wider constitutional significance! If the previous President was indeed both a frog and a puppet, he cannot possibly have been constitutionally elected. I therefore humbly request a judicial review of the result of the 1996 Election Petition which declared this Frog to be the legitimate president.'

'Splendid,' said the judge. 'Injunction granted.'

'And I also request an injunction to retroactively suspend the previous presidency, pending the outcome of the previously mentioned judicial review.'

'Never did like the little bugger,' said the Judge.

'I also seek an injunction suspending the Constitution, pending a judicial review of whether or not puppets are allowed to contest the presidency. In my view, the president is supposed to pull the strings of the other puppets, and therefore should not be a puppet himself.'

'Quite right,' said the Judge. 'I grant an injunction suspending the Constitution, pending a judicial review of whether I consider it to be sensible.'

'Furthermore,' continued Mr Surmiser, 'I surmise that members of parliament cannot have followed due process, otherwise they would not have passed such a questionable Constitution. Therefore I humbly petition this court for suspension of parliament, pending a judicial review of all MPs' bank statements.'

'What fun!' said the Judge. 'Petition granted!'

'Hey,' I said. 'Have you forgotten about me and the Cookie Monster?'

'Not at all,' said Mr Surmiser, 'I request an injunction to suspend the calendar, and to keep the date continuously at 31st July, pending the outcome of a judicial review of whether Kalaki's column can be published on 1st August.'

'Good idea,' said the Judge. 'Time stands still in my court.'

'Wake up!' shouted Sara. 'You've been asleep since the Muppet Show. You've missed the news! Judge Nyangalala has been suspended, pending a judicial enquiry!'

'I bet you didn't know,' I replied, 'that the Cookie Monster is not really a puppet. There's a real man inside that laughable costume.'

'I'm glad you've told me that,' laughed Sara.

'That's what the Frog didn't know,' I explained. 'Inside every fat man, there's a thin man struggling to get out.'

1st August 2002

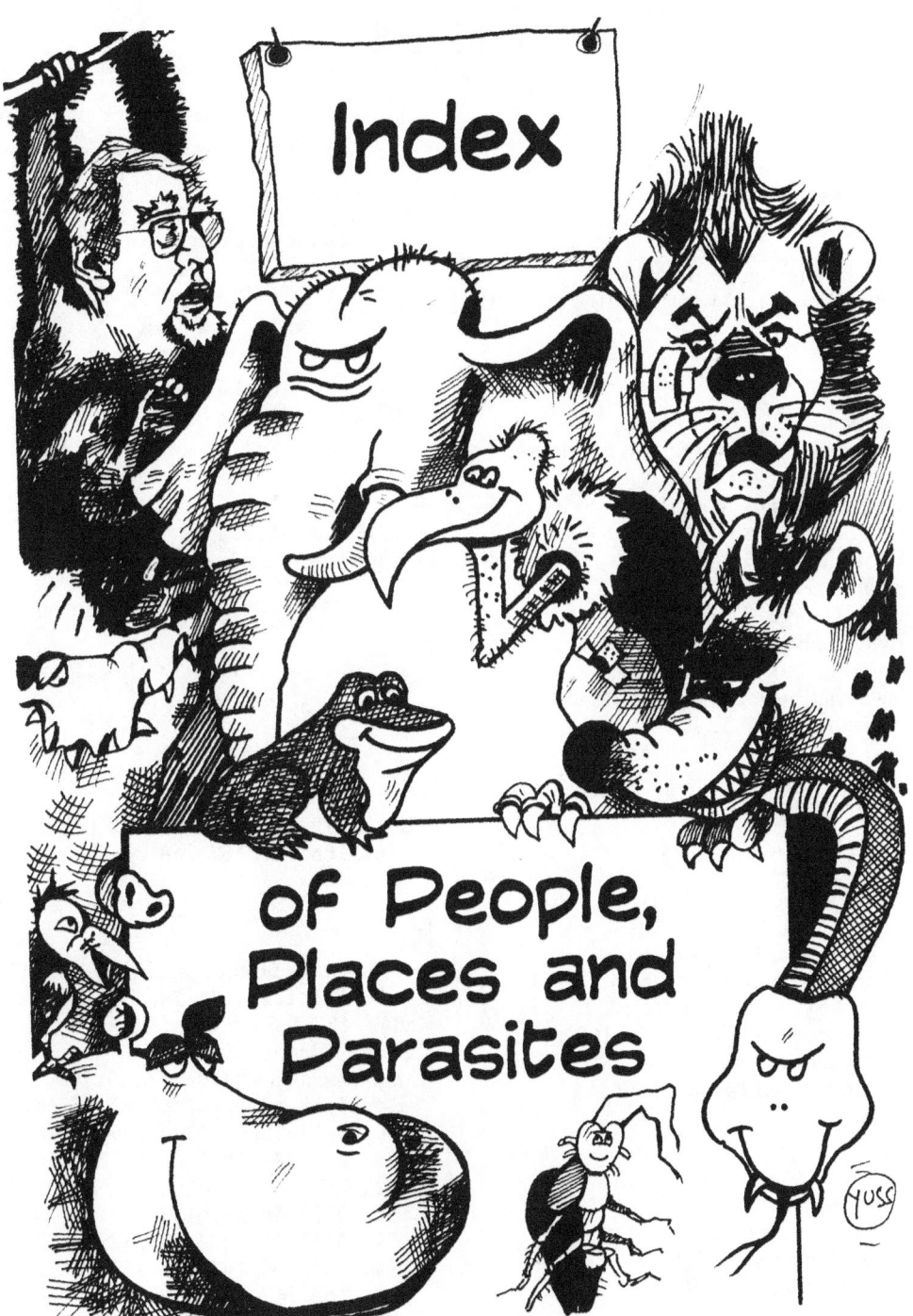

Index

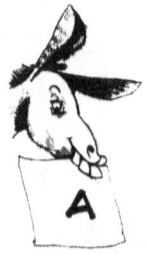

Abashi, Bigwig; 83, 163, 164
Advertisements; 74-75, 108-109, 129-130

B

Baboon; 5, 6
Bags, brown paper (see also envelopes); 127, 166
Bazooka, Randy; 85
Bling Bling, Bishop; 52, 53, 54
Boot (lickers); 108, 153
Bumble, Putrid; 5, 6
Bush, George; 47, 48
Bwalwa, Booby (see also Bwalwa, Bwamba); 65, 128, 149
Bwalwa, Bwamba (see also Bwalwa, Booby); 125, 126

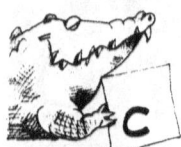

Cabbage (see also Kabeji); 22, 116, 117, 128, 140, 148, 149, 150, 151
Chabala, Charles; 150
Cherise (see also Chileshe); 152, 153
Chileshe (see also Cherise); 152, 153
Chiwelewele (various); 160, 162
Chiwelewele, Kwindi; 139, 140
Coma, Frantic; 144, 145, 146, 147

D

Dale, Penny; 17, 18
Dimba, Bedstead; 164
Dollar (anthem to); 139
Dollar (prayer to); 140

Envelopes, brown paper (see also bags); 108, 109, 153

Figov, Selloff; 81, 83
Fleddie, littul; 84, 85, 86, 87, 90, 91

G

Giraffe, knock-kneed; 2
Going, Dr Serious; 7-8

I

Indaba; 32, 33
Iscariot, Judas; 51

J

Judge(s); 13, 70, 71, 75, 97, 122-123, 160-162, 165, 166, 167, 168

K

Kabeji (see also Cabbage); 23, 25, 65, 117, 120, 121, 122, 123, 124, 127, 128
Kadoli; 46, 81, 83, 95-97
Kadopy, Valentine; 84
Kafupi (see also Wabufi); 16, 17, 18, 23, 24, 25, 28, 40, 62, 65, 66, 67, 68, 69, 70, 71, 72, 73, 74, 77, 78, 79, 87, 88, 89, 102, 103, 118, 150, 151, 165, 166
Kalaki; 8, 12, 13, 16, 18, 22, 28, 29, 46, 48, 50, 52, 55, 56, 59, 61, 75, 76, 77, 78, 79, 83, 85, 116, 124, 126, 129, 141, 144, 145, 146, 147, 152, 153, 156, 158, 165, 166, 167, 168

Kalaliki; 5, 6
Kalaliki, Laurence; 84
Kanono; 20, 22, 35, 36, 37, 122, 123
Kapinpinya, Enuch; 113-115, 117
Katendi; 35, 37, 42, 44, 45, 46, 48, 103
Kermit the Frog; 167, 168
Kondwa (Kondwani); 7, 9, 26
Konie, Dried (with Swedish sauce); 143, 148
Kupela (also Koops); 10, 11, 26, 148, 149

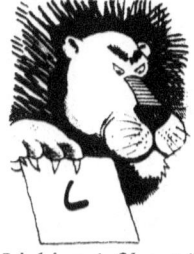

Licking (of boots); 108, 153
Luwaya; 148

M

Magistrate(s); 16, 18, 78
Makangi; 14, 15
Malambo, Villian; 20
Mango, Velvet; 68, 113, 116, 117, 122, 123, 134, 135
Mata, Cycle; 75, 95, 97, 109, 126, 151, 163, 164
Matrimony, Archie; 85
Mazoka, Steak; 143, 148, 149
Meander, Godless; 97
Meddlecraft, Sir Meddlesome; 124, 125, 126
Merry, Judge Gregarious; 160-162
Mfoola, Lazy; 32, 33
Mfuwe; 1, 2, 3, 4, 14, 15
Milungu, Archbishop; 90
Miyanda Snail (with pompous dressing); 148, 149
MMD (and all Movement for....); 2, 16, 26, 27, 38, 44, 70, 71, 108, 109, 112, 113, 116, 118, 119, 120, 124, 125, 137, 138, 140, 144, 145, 155, 160, 162, 166

M'membe, Fred; x
Morleen; 23, 25, 28, 29, 65, 75, 127, 128, 134-136, 150, 151
Mosquito, Andrew; 154, 155
Muchenjelo, Professor; 10, 11
Mulenga, Sorry; 95, 99
Mumble, Never; 50, 51
Mumbo Jumbo; 30, 31, 33, 49, 52, 54, 55, 56, 59, 60, 61
Munchishanya, Munchilinganya; 93
Munshumfwa; 27, 76, 98, 132, 144, 145, 167
Musonda, Kapelwa; ix
Muwelewele; 2, 4, 7, 9, 10, 13, 14, 15
Mwanamwanamwana; 27, 151
Mwansa, Chastity; 112
Mwelwamwelwa, Alisosa; 139, 140
Mwewa, Simon; 111
Mwinga, Jowie; ix

N

Nalumango; 42, 43
Namukolo; 106, 107, 148, 149
Ndulo, Professor Muna; 74

O

O'Flatulence, Father Fatty; 64
Orwell, George; 152

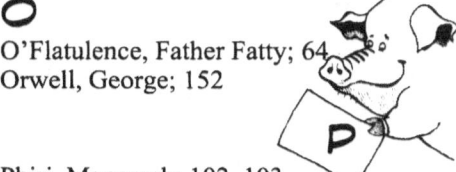

Phiri, Manasseh; 102, 103
Pilate, Pontius; 73

Q

Quakwi, Quack; 95

R

Rats; 102, 103, 106, 134, 135, 139
Regina; 66, 67
Righteous, St Simon; 90, 91
Rousseau, J.J; 120

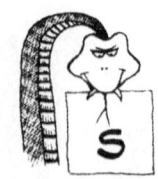

Sam; 68, 69, 93, 94, 111, 112, 137, 138, 139, 140, 154, 155, 160
Sara; 26, 27, 30, 31, 38, 39, 50, 51, 52, 54, 57, 58, 72, 77, 98, 99, 100, 101, 102, 103, 106, 107, 113, 115, 128, 132, 133, 134, 136, 148, 152, 153, 166, 168
Satan, Michael (see also Mata); 90, 91
Shikashiwa; 5, 6, 12, 13, 38, 78, 79
Shushushu; 2, 33, 65, 79, 87, 164
Sichone, Lucy; ix
Sinn, Benny; 104, 105
Snake, redlipped; 2, 7
Sofa, purple plastic; 81-83, 88, 89, 90
St Ignominious; 72, 100, 101, 132
Supple, Professor Rubble; 156, 157, 158

T

Tembo, Clismar; 90, 91
Thoko; 7, 9, 34, 38, 39, 40, 41, 42, 43
Towani; 38, 39, 41, 148

U

UNZA (see YUNZA)

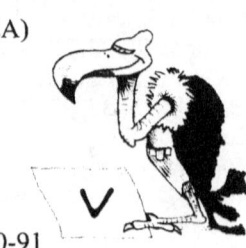

Vera; 65, 76, 77, 80-91
Vice, President of; 57, 58

W

Wabufi (Kafupi); 88, 101, 121, 128, 136
Willingo, Willy; 141, 142
Wobbly, King; 32, 33

Y

Yaliwe; 148, 149
Yumba; 38, 39, 148
YUNZA (see UNZA); 156

Z

Zulu, Oloso; 16

www.ingramcontent.com/pod-product-compliance
Lightning Source LLC
Chambersburg PA
CBHW021143230426
43667CB00005B/231